Important Numbers

Copyright © 2016 by OnlineMedEd
Edition 1.5
First published in paperback in 2015

For information about permission to use or reproduce selections from this book,
email help@onlinemeded.org with the subject, "Additional Intern Guide Usage".

Authored by Dustyn Williams
Edited by Jamie Fitch
Produced by Staci Weber

ISBN 978-0-9969501-2-1

Published by OnlineMedEd, www.onlinemeded.org

Printed in the United States of America

Dedication

To the people in my life who made this project possible.
Had it not been for them, none of this would have come to pass.

My fiancée Seeyuen Lee, for her tolerance.

My parents, Bill and Beth Williams, for their time and their faith in me.

My mentor, Chad Miller, for the advice and motivation.

My cofounder and partner, Jamie Fitch, for holding everything together.

Table of Contents

0. Prologue
   a. Introduction and disclaimer   2
   b. OnlineMedEd Story   3
   c. Tier 1 Knowledge = Topics for intern year   6
   d. On Call Pearls   7

1. Philosophy and Bureaucracy
   a. Philosophy   12
   b. Stages of Death and Dying in Residency   13
   c. Duty Hours   16
   d. The Team Cap Explained   17
   e. Morning Interdisciplinary Rounds (IDR)   18
   f. Stress   19
   g. Clinical Reasoning   20
   h. Errors in Clinical Reasoning   22
   i. Finite and Infinite Games   23
   j. Patient Satisfaction   24

2. Survival Techniques
   a. Time Management: Data Tracking   28
   b. Time Management: To Do Lists / Scut Lists   31
   c. Survival Skills: Morning Workflow   34
   d. Survival Skills: Urgent and Important   36
   e. Time Management: Turkeys and Windows   38
   f. People Management: Relationships   40
   g. People Management: Being Effective   43
   h. People Management: Arguments   44
   i. Life Management: In Your Box   46
   j. Doing Questions   47
   k. Studying Resources   48

3. Rounding and Documentation
   a. H&P: Spoken Presentation   50
   b. Daily Rounds: Spoken Presentation   52
   c. Documentation: Saying it Right (for CMS)   53
   d. H&P: Written Template   54
   e. D/C Summary: Written Template   55
   f. Ideal Admit Order Set   56
   g. Procedure Notes   58
   h. Transfer of Care / Step Down: Written Template   60

4. Medications
   a. Meds: Top 50   62
   b. Common Meds: Heart Related   64
   c. Common Meds: Lung Related   65
   d. Common Medications: Pain   66
   e. Common Meds: Poop and Vomit   67
   f. Common Medications: Psych Meds   68
   g. Antibiotics   69

5. Methods
   a. Chest Pain   72
   b. Shortness of Breath   73
   c. Abdominal Pain   74
   d. Syncope   76
   e. Weakness   77
   f. Fluid Where Fluid Shouldn't Be (Swelling)   78
   g. Delirium   79
   h. Hemoptysis   80
   i. Fever   81
   j. AKI   82
   k. Bleeding   84
   l. Dysphagia   85
   m. Back Pain   86
   n. Headache   87
   o. Joint Pain   88
   p. Diarrhea   89
   q. Pulmonary Hypertension   90
   r. ECG Interpretation   92
   s. Cough   95
   t. Acid Base and the Chamber of Secrets   96

6. Common Medical Problems
   a. Cardiac Chest Pain   102
   b. So you admitted that chest pain   103
   c. Heart Failure In the Clinic – Outpatient   104
   d. Heart Failure In the Hospital – Inpatient   105
   e. Afib   106
   f. COPD Exacerbation   107
   g. Pulmonary Embolism   108
   h. Sepsis   109
   i. Principles of Antibiotic Management   110
   j. Pneumonia   111
   k. Electrolytes - Sodium   112
   l. Electrolytes - Potassium   113
   m. Cirrhosis   114
   n. GI Bleed   119

	o.	Approach to LFTs	120
	p.	Inpatient Diabetes	121
	q.	Diabetic Ketoacidosis	122
	r.	Outpatient Diabetes	124
	s.	Stroke	125

7. Intern Notes
   - a. Cardiology — 128
   - b. Pulmonary — 131
   - c. Renal Nephrology Kidney — 134
   - d. GI and Liver — 138
   - e. Heme Onc — 141
   - f. Infectious Disease — 148
   - g. Endocrinology — 151
   - h. Rheumatology — 154
   - i. Neuro — 157

8. ICU
   - a. Sick, Not Sick, On the Fence — 160
   - b. Who Goes to the Unit? — 162
   - c. ARDS - Lung Protective Strategy — 163
   - d. Ventilator Strategy — 164
   - e. Common Medications in the ICU: Sedation and Paralysis — 166
   - f. In the ICU: Approach to Shock — 168
   - g. In the ICU: Pressors — 171
   - h. In the ICU: Septic Shock — 172
   - i. In the ICU: Running a Code — 174
   - j. In the ICU: Running a Rapid — 175

Prologue

You've come a long way.

You've much further to go.

Together we'll take on the next challenge -
your first year as a, "Real Doctor."

Train hard. Train right.

This is your playbook.

Let's make you a great physician.

REMEMBER:

"The best preparation for tomorrow is to do today's work superbly well."
– Sir William Osler

"Practice does not make perfect. Perfect practice makes perfect."
– Vince Lombardi

"Perfection is not attainable, but if we chase perfection, we will catch excellence."
– Vince Lombardi

Introduction and disclaimer

At OnlineMedEd we believe in making the hard stuff easier. Intern year is scary. We've tried to make it a little less so by building a guide that helps you with people, medicine, and most importantly, yourself. Not everything in here is evidence-based. It's yet to be tested in randomized controlled trials. Where it's been developed and vetted is in the trenches.

Using this guide, you'll get the same coaching you would as if you were training at Tulane under me. This is how I practice, coach my residents and help my students. I can't coach everyone personally, so instead I extend my playbook to you. Learn the plays, so to speak; take from it what you will and leave the rest behind.

Everything is about getting you from where you are now to where you want to be. From your point A to point B.

Again, this is how I practice. It's how I carry myself in life. It's a compilation pulling from personal experience, things I've read from people much smarter than I, and what I've been taught by people a lot better than I am. You might have a different perspective. That's ok. The opinions expressed in this book are just those. I'd like to think they're well thought out opinions, but they're opinions none the less.

I hope you enjoy this book.
I hope it makes your life better.
I hope it make you better, both as a person and as a physician.

I hope that, when the time comes, you make the right choice and help another human being. In that moment, no one will know why you did it. You may not even know why you did it. But you did. There will be no awards. No praise. No applause. There'll simply be the satisfaction that you did good for another person. Aim to be good at doing good. That's what this job is all about.

 – Dustyn

LEGAL: because it's required. This book is intended as a guide only. It is NOT intended to act as a reference book nor should it be used to replace further reading. It's not meant to be used directly for diagnoses, treatment, or patient-specific advice. It's up to you to stay current and to make choices based on the patients and the best practices. We're here to help, but don't use this as a crutch. Instead, use it as a springboard.

Also, don't steal our stuff. We make it super cheap. And we always have more. If you want to use anything in this book, write to us and let us know what you want to use it for. We'll probably say yes.

OnlineMedEd Story

The origin story of OnlineMedEd is one that's all too typical. Ever sit in class and find yourself thinking, "Why are they making this so much harder than it needs to be?" Yep, me too. Med school is hard. Med schools make med school harder. Perhaps there's logic; as hard as it was, the experience of medical school forged who I am, how I practice, and how I teach. But as I found a way to survive, I became resolute in finding a better way for those that followed.

I found that medical students succeed in spite of the curriculum, not because of it. Let's just say I wasn't a happy person in the first two years of medical school. I contributed a lot to Tulane, helping rebuild it after Hurricane Katrina. I even won a few awards. I don't tell you this to brag; I do this because even though I was successful, I suffered. Mentally and emotionally – this wasn't the way it was supposed to be. I went to medical school to help people; what happened?

By the time third year rolled around I finally had enough. A flash point moment drove me to start making videos. During my Ob/Gyn rotation I sat down for a two-hour lecture. There were eight of them in the block. Eight lectures. This one was entitled, "contraception." I walked in thinking, *"I don't know much about contraception other than what I see on TV."* This was before rings, implants and packets had flooded cable. In that two-hour lecture I was lectured on every nuance of every pill. It was separated by dose of estrogen, progesterone, and the fudge factor (how forgiving a missed pill was). That was it – two hours of oral contraceptive discussion only. I left thinking, *"I don't know much about contraception other than what I see on TV."* The answer on the shelf was "OCPs".

To his credit, the lecturer was an excellent speaker. He was also a reproductive endocrinologist; he taught what's important to him. It would have been extremely valuable if we were reproductive endocrinology fellows. But we were 3rd year medical students, 6 years away from that fellowship, and most of us weren't going into Ob/Gyn.

I don't fault him; he's not paid to teach. He likely was never taught how to do it either. Given little direction or training, it's easy to understand why he taught what he wanted, rather than what the students needed to learn. This moment caused me to ask myself: What do I want? What does everyone else want? What do they need? Why aren't they teaching to that specifically? Everyone has a finite time in medical school. There's too much to know to try to learn it all.

It's really about the foundation, the basics. Medical information grows at an exponential rate; specialists exist for a reason. You can't learn everything about everything. You'll learn the details of your specialty in residency and beyond. Those 4 years have nothing to do with that.

That's what no one seemed to realize, or at least do much to address.

So I went to work to change that. I got a white board, a camera, and a cameraman (my girlfriend). The first lectures were so bad and boring she fell asleep while filming me. I built the website myself; it wasn't much better.

But people watched. More people came and the first people came back again and again.

No matter how bad those first lectures were, I realized they were better than what most students were getting. After countless hours of practice and some formal training in education, the videos turned the corner. First medicine, then surgery, peds, ob, neuro, psych. The videos kept coming; I got better (some you may still find some of the old ones… they're still bad).

That's when Jamie, a clinical epidemiologist and friend that had seen the whole thing, challenged me to think bigger. The videos were good, but the site wasn't. People wanted the knowledge, but so few knew about them. Why not create a platform that could promote and sustain itself, and offer more to more people? He offered to help, joined me, and took the site to the next level. To achieve our goals we developed a mechanism to grow, share, and draw more students in.

What we strive for now is to help people. As doctors, of course, but also as educators and people.

Medical knowledge belongs to no one; it should be accessible to everyone. Now, anyone with an internet connection can get the basics of medical knowledge. They can learn how to practice. Bringing that to the world is one of the most inspiring things about this company and this site. We're not about turning a profit, or making a sale. We're about bringing more people more access to more knowledge than ever before at a global level.

People caught on and were inspired. They began volunteering to help with content; I was shocked. Why would someone I don't know, have never met, do something for me and my website and insist on not being paid for their work?

Then one guy told me: OnlineMedEd gives willingly and saves people from the same bitterness and frustration that I felt back in that contraceptives lecture. We give, so others give back.

Today, the community grows. The site grows. The content grows. The vision is to have a place where anyone at any point in their training can go to learn what's needed for their level. And it's happening.

This is where you come in. Likely, you're not reading this because you heard the Online-MedEd Intern Guide was so awesome you had to have it, but because you've been with us through it all. It isn't sexy. But what it's got is soul.

It may not look pretty, but if it helps you help someone else, that's all we care about. As you grow with this site you'll see it grow with you.

What I really want to say is thanks. One, for reading through three pages of fluff. Two, for caring enough about your patients and your team to be willing to carry this guide around. Whatever you think your reason is for holding onto this book is, there's only one reason you're here: to help people.

We'll help you help people. We can show you the way. You have to take the path and go on this journey. We can't bring you from point A to point B, but we sure can light up some signs for you along the way.

Continue to grow. Continue to get better.

One day, you'll be responsible for a human life. Without supervision, without help, you'll do for others. Maybe you'll teach.

And that's really why I say thanks.

Carry on the legacy: help others to help others all the while helping others.

Sincerely,

Dustyn Williams, MD

Tier 1 Knowledge = Topics for intern year

1. Diabetes
2. Anemia
3. Potassium
4. Sodium
5. Acute Renal Failure
6. Acid Base
7. Asthma / COPD
8. Pneumonia
9. GI Bleed
10. Antibiotics
11. Meningitis
12. HIV = Opportunistic Infections and PPX
13. CHF Exacerbation
14. CHF Clinic
15. Afib / Aflutter
16. Chest Pain / Coronary Artery Disease
17. Shock = Differential
18. Shock = Pressors
19. Shock = Resuscitation
20. Altered Mental Status
21. Thrombocytopenia
22. Alcohol Withdrawal
23. Tachycardia
24. Syncope
25. Hepatitis
26. Weakness
27. Bradycardia
28. Liver Enzyme Assessment
29. Sickle Cell Anemia
30. Thyroid Disorders

On Call Pearls

Constipation
Lactulose 30 ml PO qD
Dulcolax
Milk of Magnesia 60 ml PO
Colace 50-100 mg qD

Diarrhea
Lomotil 10 ml PO qD
Imodium 4 mg PO x 1
- Then 2 mg after each episode (16 mg/d max)

Nausea/Vomiting
Phenergan 12.5/25 mg PO/IV q6h, 4 mg IVP
Zofran 4mg IV over 2-5 mins, or 4 mg IM

Dry Eyes
Natural Tears 1-2 drops QHS TID or QID

Hypotension
Stop HTN meds
NS or LR 250 ml-500 ml bolus
Stat H/H
Type and screen 2 units if unsure
Type and cross 2 units if sure
    Tylenol 650 mg 30 mins before transfusion
    Benadryl 25 mg PO 30 mins before transfusion
    Post transfusion CBC in 6 hours

Shock
EKG + CXR + H/H
Pressor Dopamine 5 mcg/kg/min
    Titrate to systolic >100 MAP >60, max of 20 mcg/km/min
Levophed 8-12 mcg/min . Maintenance 2-4 mcg/min

Hematuria
Clots? / Pink?
Stop Heparin, NOT Coumadin
PT/PTT/INR
3-way Foley
Continuous Bladder irrigation with 3L free H2O

Agitation
Access reason, telemetry monitor?
Orient
Ativan 1 mg IV x1
Haldol 5 mg IM q4h PRN (geriatrics)

Pain
Lortab 5-10 mg PO
Percocet 5-10 mg PO
Morphine 2-4 mg IV x 1
Dilaudid 1 mg IV x 1 (0.5 if pt is frail)

SOB
Sats? Liters?
Titrate nasal cannula 5-6 liters to > 90%
Nasal Cannula
Ventimask
Non-rebreather
Bipap (CHF/COPD): 50% 02, 12 Inspir & 6 Expir cm H20
Albuterol and Atrovent nebs = Duonebs
Xopenex if pt has persistent tachycardia
Lasix if wet (double dose of PO as IV form)
    Get CXR, ABG, EKG, CBC/BMP
If sudden aspiration, ask Resp. Therapy to deep suction

Post Op Fever
Expect Post Op Fever in pt's s/p Ortho procedures
Don't draw cultures, give Tylenol, unless POD >7

HTN
Clonidine 0.2 mg PO x 1
    PO q4h PRN SBP >160 DBP >100
    Max. 0.5-0.7/day
Lopressor 5 mg IV x 1
Labetalol IV 10-20 mg x 1 (if they don't tolerate PO)
    Cardiac monitor
Nitropaste 2 in to anterior chest wall
Hydralazine 5 mg IVP x 1

Hypokalemia
KCl 40 meq PO (K Dur)
KCL 40 meq + 250 ml NS over 4 hours (aka K Ryder)
Never >10 meq/h—it burns
If K+ < 3, K-Dur 40 meq PO + Ryder 40 meq IV
Each 10 meq increases K+ by 0.1

Hypomagnesemia
MagOx x TID iflow Mg
Magnesium 2 g IV over 1 hour

Hyperkalemia
Kayexalate 60 g PO q 6h PRN
Calcium gluconate 1 amp
Insulin 10 units + D50 1 amp

Vancomycin Trough
If Vanc trough <20, can give Vanc Dose

Cough
Tessalon perles 100 mg PO q8h prn

Itching
Hydroxyzine 25-50 mg po q6-8h PRN
Benadryl 25-50 mg po q6-8h PRN

GI prophylaxis
Should be done with H2 blockers bid
Burn patients
Head injury
Full Dose anticoagulation
On Vent for > than 48 hours
Chronic Medications such as anti-inflammatories, Steroids
Otherwise, there is NO indication for GI prophylaxis

To Pronounce a death
Check pupils, heartbeat, chest rise, breath sounds, give vigorous sterna rub, pulses.

Sample Death Note:
Nurse name paged me to examine pt at time. Pt. Unresponsive, even to painful stimuli,
Pupils fixed & non reactive. Pt has no spontaneous breathing, no heart sounds or breath
sounds. No carotid, or femoral pulses present. No heart sounds or breath sounds heard.
Time of death pronounced at time on date.

Family Notified by (myself or nurse).
Grievance services offered to family.
Body to be released to funeral home of family's choice.

Philosophy
and
Bureaucracy

The principles by which to live one's life

&

The rules that confine your soul.

Do well at doing good.

Inspire yourself, inspire others.

Keep yourself safe, keep others safe.

"In seeking absolute truth we aim at the unattainable
and must be content with broken portions."
— *Sir William Osler*

CHAPTER 1: PHILOSOPHY AND BUREAUCRACY

Philosophy

1. **Show up** – mentally and physically; be ready to take care of patients and to learn. It's not about checking the boxes and getting through the day. It's about engaging, trying, succeeding, failing, and growing. That can't happen if you aren't here.

2. **Be honest** – you're in control of the team and the patients. You know the details and the data. If you lie, no one will catch you, but the patient will suffer. If you don't know, just say as much. There are consequences for not doing what you are supposed to. Those consequences are far less than a lie that harms another human being.

3. **Play as a team** – this is 80 hours a week, 48 weeks a year, for 3 years of your life. You aren't an employee; you're a team member. These are your friends and teammates; they're your life every day, in and out. Teams win when they play together.

The above three must be given precedence over all others. They're the golden rules. With them, your life will be fulfilling. Without them, no one can trust you; pain and misery will be felt. Those that follow are valuable, but the ones above are necessary.

4. **Practice** – the only way to get good at seeing patients is to see patients. However, remember that practice doesn't make perfect; perfect practice makes perfect. Make it count.

5. **Make decisions** – growth comes from failure, not success. Failure comes from trying. Make a decision. Stick by it. Find out if you were right or wrong. Come to rounds with that decision and ask for feedback; don't come waiting to be told what to do.

6. **Build methods, be methodical** – develop methods to help yourself and your patients. Stick by them. The more you practice good methods, the more innate they become. Yes, it's more work up front. But, it pays in spades on the back end.

7. **Read** – there are things you need to know that you may never see. To know about them you must read and learn about them. Pick whichever book you want, but read. See Survival Techniques and Study resources. You can also just watch OnlineMedEd.

8. **Teach** – teaching will help you learn what you don't know. It'll also teach your learners what you do know. Passing on the gift of knowledge is part of the right of passage from student to master.

9. **Live** – take the time to do something good for yourself. Love someone or something. Go fishing. Go biking. Go to the club. Maintain the passions that make you who you are. Share them with the team. These are your friends and kin for the next three years.

STAGES OF DEATH AND DYING IN RESIDENCY

Stages of Death and Dying in Residency

Remember the Kübler-Ross stages of death and dying from Psych? Well get ready - you're about to go through them in residency. Like stages of death and dying, you can oscillate between them in a variety of orders.

Remember, it turns out that literally **everyone before you has gone through this already**. There are plenty of people to turn to for help: your mentors (faculty), friends (co-interns), and team (upper levels). I can't stress this enough – we've all been there. You're not alone.

1. Denial (actually fear)

You're here, so it's too late for denial. Rather, what most people manifest isn't denial; it's fear. I'M A DOCTOR! I'M HERE! I'M READY! (not denial). Then it sinks in. "Damn, I'm a doctor, but I'm not ready…"

You're a newly minted doctor. Your name now means something. You can sign orders and write notes. Chances are you also haven't done **anything medicine related since your Sub-I a year ago**. Some people walk into residency and think, "great, time to warm up." Then they're handed seven brand new patients and a pager. Go.

That can and likely will be terrifying. But with experience (and this guide) you'll garner the skills required to handle twice that. You just need some pointers and some practice.

But there's something else that eats away at you - the **charlatan**. EVERYONE knows that you're new and don't know anything - you're just a student in disguise. The fear of being "caught" or having your secret revealed can weigh heavily on the soul. You're supposed to be the team leader and exude confidence, but how is that possible when everyone knows you're a fake?

These are **good feelings**. It means you're humble. It means you fear hurting your patients. They're **normal**. Embrace them; the fear and excitement you fret over now will turn into exhilaration in a few months.

2. Depression

You've been chugging along pretty well. You're finally used to the wards, the EMR, and the system. You know where you need to be and what you need to do. You have your data tracker, scutt-list (see survival skills), and have been grinding 80 hour weeks (averaged over a month). 1 Day off in 7. At least you're getting paid! (sort of)

But then it happens. Remember in school when you went through a semester of constant grinding? It ended with a big test followed by a TWO WEEK BREAK. That's what we called "winter recess." It was a great time to recharge and recalibrate. Well, guess what? There ain't no winter recess no more!

13

CHAPTER 1:   PHILOSOPHY AND BUREAUCRACY

Now, for the first time in 4 years you hit a wall. The hours start to drag, the lack of sleep begins to take hold, and the constant demands everyone has of you become draining. It's more and more challenging to keep up with all the tasks. *The patients, the nurses, the upper levels, the attendings… oh and Step 3… oh and evaluations… oh and procedure logs… ah right and I have to do that poster…* When your mind is begging for a recharge, none comes. Maybe you're at a program like mine where we got a week off on the holidays. Lucky you. If you're not given the time off, it can be even worse.

Just remember who you are and why you did this. Keep something of yourself in residency (your cat, weight lifting, pistol competition, reading fantasy novels starring Dorian Grey). But most importantly, remember why you chose to do this: **to mend the wounded, heal the sick, and comfort the dying**. You can always take solace knowing this is the best mission on the planet. No one else can say they contribute to the world as much as you do.

If you stay here for too long, **get help**. Everyone has a bad day, a really rough call, a miss, and maybe even an unintentional death. Being upset at a failure or a particularly brutal day isn't bad – it shows you care. It's when you don't bounce back that it's an issue and time to talk to someone. I don't mean get on pills; I mean talk to your mentor, the program director, or tell a friend. You'll never know where the solution will come from.

3. Bargaining

"How did I get myself into this!? Maybe I can still get out."

Bargaining comes in two forms:

The first is literal bargaining. You go to SDN.net and post for a change of residency. You're ready to give up on it. Now, if you're in a truly abusive environment or suffering real clinical depression, it's time to get out. But otherwise bailing on the team isn't the way to do it. Every place has their problems - the "stuff" that is done poorly or the "stuff" that can and should change. Every place has their awesome too. It'll be different "stuff" at different places, but the depression and bargaining will likely remain. A change of venue won't help.

The second is figurative bargaining. *Let me get through this call; THEN I can really recharge.* Be careful with this thought process. If you start coming in just to check boxes to get through the day, or worse - you start paying people to cover shifts - you're going to suffer in the long run. A much needed long sleep or a golden weekend with friends does wonder. But take those as they come. Don't compromise your training or yourself. Never give up on excellence.

STAGES OF DEATH AND DYING IN RESIDENCY

4. Anger

So you've figured it out; this intern thing is beat. You're ready to be a resident and you know it. Or, it's half way through second year and you have this resident thing down too. You don't need any more training. But that attending is STILL telling you what to do.

I know how the game works. I really wish that nurse from 4A would stop calling me every twenty minutes. LOOK AT THE DAMN CHART FIRST. No, case manager, I actually don't know, nor do I care, whether this person meets inpatient or obs - isn't that your job? Wait, I have to fill out this nursing home form AGAIN because YOU screwed it up? The system is broken, people suck, and everyone is bringing me down.

Yep, welcome to the anger stage. Here it's imperative to be REALLY careful. If you've spent your intern year depositing into emotional bank accounts (see survival skills), you've built strong relationships. But when you're angry you'll take HUGE withdrawals from everyone. You won't even know you're doing it. You'll lose allies, or worse, create enemies. Those with a robust emotional account you can probably keep, but those whom you've given few or no deposits turn on you. The result will be compromising relationships with everyone you need.

Step back and take a breath. Recognize what's in your box, your sphere of influence. You can't fix Epic and you can't get your program to change from Paragon to something else. You can't control that Nurse on 4A or that jerk attending that won't stop riding you. Even though you feel pretty damn secure right now, just realize there's always something for you to know, and something to learn from each person the stokes the bitter fire of anger.

5. Acceptance.

This is where you want to be. It's the nirvana of training. Nothing bothers you; you accept the inefficiencies for what they are and develop workarounds. You don't mind the three-charts-at-once-with-half-worked-up-patients-from-the-terrible-ED-resident-at-3 AM.

You don't mind because you've identified what you're good at, what you're not, what you can control, and what you can't. You influence where you can influence and just deal with the rest. No system is perfect. The one you're in sure isn't. The one you move to won't be either. But that's ok, you don't mind.

You'll go in and out of these phases. The goal is to reach acceptance and stay there. Believe me, when you're there you'll know. You won't bitch about the hours, the nurse on 5 center, or even the workload in front of you. You'll look forward to coming into the hospital. You'll go with the flow and be flexible. When you reach this point, you've gained enough skill and agility to work around most obstacles. Your attendings will see it and you'll take yet another step forward to being the best you can be.

CHAPTER 1: PHILOSOPHY AND BUREAUCRACY

Duty Hours

Duty hours are a hot topic. We want you to be safe. And by that I mean mentally, emotionally, and physically safe. You need to eat. You need to sleep. If you want to, you need to work out / pet your dog / pet your lover / whatever you need to do to decompress your soul. AND... We want you to practice safe medicine for our patients.

BUT...

You're here to learn. Be focused on learning the medicine, the business, and yes... doing the work. By work... I mean, of course, writing the notes (ugh).

So to help you keep your eye on the prize, it's important to better understand duty hours.

No more than 80 hours per week in a 4 week period. *That's an average.*
That means, technically, you have 320 hours in 4 weeks to work. That DOES NOT MEAN 80 hours a week. It means if you work 72 hours one week, it's ok to work 88 the next. I know it sucks to work the 88 hours that week, but it is ok for you to stay an hour or two for necessary transitions, sick patients, or to grab that procedure you really want. We do everything to get you out way below 80, but I want you to see that if you WANT to stay to get something out of that time you CAN.

"1 day off in 7" in a 4 week period. *That's an average.*
That means, technically, you have 4 days in 4 weeks that you must have off. A "day off" means 24 hours between "shifts." I hate that word. You don't work shifts. You're not a postal worker; you're a doctor. You don't even work; you practice an art. You know what I mean... but I digress.

We try to get you one day off a week, usually a weekend, where you leave the night before and don't come back until the morning after. Like, 36 hours off. That's the goal anyway. And we try to do it every week. This should never be an issue for you.

Interns 16 hours in a row, then an 8 hour break.
This means 16 hours in the hospital. It's mandatory work that you must do and be present for. There's a HUGE grey zone here. Your notes were supposed to be written by 4pm. You were supposed to do that discharge summary within 24 hours. But you went home. Now it's 10pm and you're finishing them from bed (please don't do this - get them done before you leave). Does THAT count as duty hours? No.

You're obsessive-compulsive / neurotic / care too much / whatever and are stalking your patient at midnight on Paragon from your phone while getting a drink with your significant other (please don't do this either). Does THAT count as duty hours? No.

Take the grey out of it; stay at the hospital until all your work is done. Don't stay longer than 15 hours. FIFTEEN. That way you leave at fifteen and don't come anywhere close to 16.

THE TEAM CAP EXPLAINED

The Team Cap Explained

Understanding residency limits can be hard, but it's important as you should know when you're about to reach yours. Going over the limit doesn't matter for "violations." It matters because you're here to learn and take care of patients. Yes, you need patient volume to do so. Yes, more patients will force you to learn to get faster and more efficient. BUT... we want you learning, not working. We want you SAFELY taking care of patients, not hurting them. Hence, there's a necessity for caps.

1. A **new admit** is a patient that you get the call for. The beeper goes off. It's you and the ED. You see the patient, write the H&P. You put in the admit orders. You do everything – it's your patient.

2. A **consult** is a patient admitted to someone else that you facilitate medical management for. This is frustrating because ACGME DOESN'T see this as a new admit. In fact, consults don't count for anything, which we think is a little silly. Consider a consult like you would a new admit. You're going to see the patient, write an H&P, and follow every day. Count it towards your team cap even though you and I know ACGME doesn't count it.

3. A **transfer** is anything else: night float admits that are given to your team the next morning, ICU step-downs that you weren't already following, or a surgery patient that surgery doesn't want to take care of anymore. Whatever the case may be it's an already admitted patient that you now take care of. Where this gets tricky is with patients from the ED during the morning. If a pit boss admits to you AND does the H&P, it's a transfer. If YOU do the H&P, it's an admit.

4. A **patient contact** is any patient seen. This means new admits, consults, transfers, old patients, whatever. There's NO LIMIT to the number of patient contacts.

The **CAP** is based on **continuing care** patients. That means patients that stay on your service. It's counted when you go home for the day. The number of patients LEFT ON YOUR SERVICE AT THE END OF THE DAY THAT YOU'LL SEE TOMORROW is your **census.**

If census is greater than cap, that's bad.

Census > CAP = Bad

If patient contacts are greater than your cap, all is well.

Contacts > CAP = OK

A <u>resident </u>can have 14 new patients in a call cycle [7am-7pm for us].
- 10 new admits, transfers, consults (our rule), or supervising an intern on new patients
- + 4 transfers

An <u>intern </u>can have 7 new patients in a call cycle [7am-7pm for us].
- 5 new admits, consults (our rule), or transfers
- +2 transfers

A <u>team </u>can have 14 new patients in a call cycle.
- 10 new admits or transfers   1-Resident, 2-Intern team has a CAP of **20**
- +4 transfers   1-Resident, 1-intern team has a CAP of **14**

CHAPTER 1: PHILOSOPHY AND BUREAUCRACY

Morning Interdisciplinary Rounds (IDR)

This IS NOT about medical decision making. This is NOT about the disease. This is NOT about the team. This is NOT about you.

YOU WILL GET NOTHING OUT OF MORNING IDR

Morning Interdisciplinary Rounds are for <u>everyone NOT the MD team</u>. It's a place for social work, physical therapy, and case management. You have to put yourself in the mindset of the case managers (observation vs inpatient), social workers (what discharge needs are there and when can we get started?), and the PT/OT/ST people (where can these patients go after they discharge?)

Everyone (other than you) should leave the room having personally answered these three questions for themselves:
- "What do I need to do today?"
- "Is the person being discharged?"
- "Do I need anything in particular from the MD team to get my job done?"

DO
1. **Be Brief:** "64 year old lady, cap pneumonia" is all you have to say.
2. If **being discharged** say, "discharging." If there's a possibility, say, "maybe home today."
3. If you **need something** say, "needs [thing you need]" (PICC, Home Health, SNF eval).
4. If the discharge is contingent on something, tell everyone what that thing is so everyone can help get it done (consults, stress test, getting a cab, calling the police, etc).
5. **Ask about plastic.** Nursing should come with this: Foley's, Central Lines, NG Tubes, and IV fluids. If someone has one, ask if they still need it. Do this every day until that patient doesn't have it anymore.
6. **Confirm DVT prophylaxis.** It's the hottest topic right now in hospital medicine.

DO NOT
1. Linger
2. Give an overnight event recap or explain what's happened during the hospital stay.
3. Start talking about anything related to the medicine (antibiotics, pressors, etc)

This is hard. The DO NOT is literally everything you do. It's YOUR mindset and what YOU think is important. Plus, you're ready to talk about it on rounds with your attending, so you've been mentally preparing it. **News flash – you don't matter**; IDR is for ancillary staff, not for you.

Since you're thinking like your staff and team members, it's a great opportunity to make a deposit in their emotional bank account. If you walk in demanding from them, it's a withdrawal and IDR will rarely profit anything for YOU. Its rewards, however, can be abundant if you think like them, help them with their work, and make them feel important.

Stress

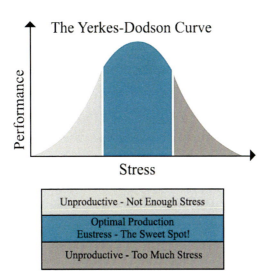

When the learner **isn't stressed at all** that is called **boredom**. When bored, the learner won't grow.

When the learner is **stressed too much** they'll enter **survival mode**. Here, the learner will put survival skills into use (see survival skills chapter) to make it through the day, but won't grow.

If the learner is given **just enough stress** they'll feel it as **eustress**. THIS IS GOOD. It's the right amount of pressure where the learner is motivated. They feel that energy to not only get the work done, but to do it well. They are forced just outside their comfort zone, pushed right up to breaking, but not over the edge. Here, the learner will grow and improve.

It's my personal belief that **eustress occurs at 12-15 patients for a 1-resident 2-intern team**. There are enough patients to be seen where there isn't down time, enough patients on service to have a wide breadth of disease experience. There are here also few enough patients so that there's time to talk about each patient in enough detail (and maybe even time for a chalk talk!).

This is why we recommend capping resident teams at 16 patients. If there are others, we just have the attendings see those themselves.

[Note: in the team cap section, we provide the ACGME CAPS of 20 and 14. I think team caps for internal medicine should be 16 (1Res-2Int) and 12 (1Res-1Int)]

CHAPTER 1:   PHILOSOPHY AND BUREAUCRACY

Clinical Reasoning

Clinical reasoning is about taking a **chief complaint** (nebulous, vague, uncertain) and turning it into a **diagnosis** (concrete, certain, specific). It's the hardest thing to do in medicine and the singular skill that separates great physicians from the good ones.

A person who has **MASTERED CLINICAL REASONING**, the only skill that separates the physician from every other employee in health care, follows this pattern:

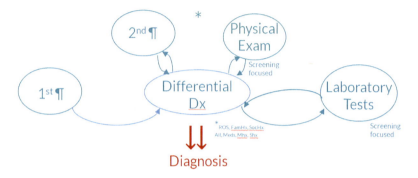

It begins with the **chief complaint**. From there, it's about ascertaining the **timing and characterization** of the disease. At Tulane, I teach **FARCOLDER** (<u>F</u>requency, <u>A</u>ssociated <u>S</u>ymptoms, <u>R</u>adiation, <u>C</u>haracter, <u>L</u>ocation, <u>D</u>uration, <u>E</u>xacerbating factors, <u>R</u>elieving factors). Do this for **every patient every time**. It becomes the **first paragraph** of every H&P. From the timing and characterization of the disease, screen that information through your brain. That filter comes up with a **differential diagnosis**. Use **methods** and **approaches** to come up with a **long list** based on the complaint. Take that information gleaned from the first paragraph to narrow it down to a "**smart list**." Have 3-5 options.

Using the smart list as a guide, ask a review of system questions that increases or decreases the pretest probability of everything on the differential. The history drives the differential, which in turn drives the question you ask. They'll be different for each patient, but will be the same for each differential each time. This is the **second paragraph** of the H&P. It influences and rearranges the order of the diagnoses on the smart list, making some more and others less likely.

The physical exam comes after this new differential. The **tier I exam** is done for every patient every time. It's the screening exam: do it regardless of the problem. After all, if the patient's sick enough to be admitted to the hospital, they are sick enough to warrant a head-to-toe exam. The differential does drive the **tier II exam**, where specific exam maneuvers performed to increase or decrease the pretest probability of the differential (JVD for Heart failure, for example). In turn, it influences the smart list like the second paragraph did.

CLINICAL REASONING

From there you order some labs and arrive a diagnosis.

Notice that? Labs are an afterthought. They're where novices go first, but are actually the least useful. We need labs and imaging as a society and as a medical system. But labs shouldn't be a starting point; they're to confirm what you've already decided. Labs too have Tier I, screening labs (CBC, BMP) and **Tier II, diagnostic labs**. These Tier II labs will influence the smart list. Hopefully they'll allow you to conclude on one diagnosis to treat.

Out the bottom comes the **diagnosis** to be treated.

What if I still don't know the diagnosis?

1. Two diagnoses that both fit

Consider the **treatment threshold**. To do so, think STEP (Safety, Tolerability, Efficacy, and Price). The more STEP something is, the less certain you have to be to give it. For example, oxygen isn't without risk, but putting a nasal cannula on 95% of patients will likely do no harm. At the other end of the spectrum is chemotherapy. It's extremely toxic, which necessitates that you're 100% sure of the diagnosis before giving it. If two competing diagnoses have each crossed the treatment threshold, treat both. You make up the number – how sure you need to be to treat, how sure you are that they have this diagnosis – but it's ok to treat two things at once.

2. Therapeutics as Diagnostics

Sometimes the treatment for one will worsen the other. So **make big moves**. Aren't sure if they're volume overloaded or volume down? Give a ton of fluid. If they get hypoxemic, they were wet. If they improve, you were right - they were dry. OR, give LARGE doses of Lasix. If their creatinine bumps they were dry; if they diurese and improve they were wet. Therapeutics and the response to them can be used to gauge whether or not you have the right diagnosis. But if you use this strategy, don't piddle. Make **big moves** to be certain of the direction they swing.

3. Get more tests / Ask more questions / do more physical exams

Sometimes the diagnosis isn't certain and something else must be done to figure it out. That's ok. Also, the ED's job isn't to make a diagnosis; it's to stabilize and triage. The person sending a direct admit from their clinic just knows they're sick. YOUR job is to make the diagnosis. Never accept the diagnosis the ED gives you. Do it yourself from scratch to assure they're right!

CHAPTER 1: PHILOSOPHY AND BUREAUCRACY

Errors in Clinical Reasoning

The novice must employ **analytical reasoning** because there's been insufficient experience to "feel" a diagnosis. Every piece of information might be important; each is carefully calculated to determine whether the differential diagnosis is right or wrong.

More experienced physicians employ **intuitive reasoning** - that is, they react. They've had sufficient experience to "smell the MI" or "hear the cellulitis calling." This comes with thousands of patients and tens of thousands of hours of experience.

The best physicians utilize **intuitive reasoning**, but are also savvy enough to know when "something isn't right" and know how and when to employ **analytical reasoning**.

The weakest physicians overly rely on **intuitive reasoning**, using only pattern-recognition to guide them. Nurses can do this. PAs can do this. They're often right, but not always. As physicians we must do more.

> Both **analytical reasoning** and **intuitive reasoning** are good things. It's essential to know when to use one over the other. You don't have the experience yet. Rely on analytical reasoning now, so you develop the right intuition. CONCIOUSLY REFLECT on how and what you do.

Anchoring:
The most dangerous of all errors is anchoring. This is when you prematurely close on a diagnosis and ignore all other information that's counter to your decision. Each intervention, lab, and diagnostic test is another data point. In anchoring, the PE gets admitted as CHF, 6 times (this happened). Only when analytical reasoning was employed did I (Dustyn) diagnose a PE in a guy who had been admitted over and over for CHF (not by Dustyn).

Recency Heuristic (formally called Availability Heuristic)
This happens when you just saw something in another patient and allow it to become more likely in THIS patient. Each patient must be considered in isolation of all other patients. Things do not "come in threes." It's more likely you're you making a reasoning error.

Severity:
"We have to rule out PE because it's so deadly." So is smallpox. How many times have you ruled out smallpox for a rash? More deadly doesn't mean more likely. The ED is most often guilty of this.

Confirmation Bias (i.e. Consultant-Said-So Bias)
Just because the ED says it's pneumonia does not mean it is. That said, if you go on their word you'll find the evidence that supports it (this parallels Anchoring). Go the other way and draw your own conclusions. It might happen to be the same - great! But don't let someone else blindly tell you what the diagnosis is. Yes, not even your attendings (unless they back it up).

Finite and Infinite Games

In your career to date you've been playing **finite games**. They have a start time, a stop time, rules on how to play, and rules on how to win. That was the shelf, the USMLE Step 2, the grade, and graduation. When playing finite games you have a role and see others as playing their role. But people are not roles. They are people. They have feelings, emotions, and souls. Finite games crush people, and your "win" is often someone else's loss.

Hopefully you developed survival skills. You might have "beaten the game" by figuring out what had to be done to get the A, the honors. And that's great, because you survived. But now, more importantly than any point in your career, it's time stop playing finite games and start playing infinite ones. The grade doesn't matter. People matter.

Yes, residency has a start and end point, a set of rules, and a test to wrap it up - JUST LIKE WHAT YOU'VE DONE YOUR WHOLE LIFE. Yes, you can continue to play a finite game and "win." Pass the test, get through residency, and check the box.

You'll see people still in that mindset. They're the ones avoiding consults, writing crap notes, and treating people poorly. They'll do the bare minimum to "win." They'll focus on MKSAP17 and only care about what's "on the boards."

You **don't want to be this person**. They WON'T be effective. And they will be miserable.

In **infinite games** there are no end points, no winners, and no losers. These games don't have roles – they have people. It's the game you must now learn to play. If you haven't played this way before, yes it will be challenging. But, it's a transition you must make.

Never again will you have as much support, supervision, and feedback as in residency. You will develop more in these three years than you have in your entire life so far. Never again will you grow this much. You get a taste of autonomy. Your signature matures. Your notes carry weight. YOU matter. You will be forced to learn things you never wanted to learn. You will take care of people you don't want to take care of. But you'll grow.

THIS IS THE TIME TO LEARN and become **EFFECTIVE**. This game lasts the rest of your life. Now can't be a time in life that you, "just get through to see the other side."

- See people as people with emotions, souls, egos, and fears. You'll be effective.
- See patients as people with emotions, souls, egos, and fears. You'll be effective.
- See learners as people with emotions, souls, egos, and fears. You'll be effective.

The more effective you become during training, the more effective you will be in life. You won't rise to some superhuman ability upon graduation; you'll be reduced to your basest form of training. The further you rise, the more you learn, the better you are and the more effective you become now, the better you'll be for the rest of your life.

There is no winning or losing in residency– there's only effectiveness in patient care.

CHAPTER 1: PHILOSOPHY AND BUREAUCRACY

Patient Satisfaction

You'll hear a lot of things from a variety of people, including many bureaucrats and administrators trying to get their HCAHPS ("HCAP") scores up. That doesn't have anything to do with pneumonia; it's about patient satisfaction. If you've read anything in this philosophy section you know it has nothing to do with, "stating medication side effects," or, "explaining the diagnosis to the family." You get good patient satisfaction scores by connecting on a human level (who would have guessed?).

The problem is that everything we've discussed so far is about creating relationships, particularly long-lasting ones where trust is built over time. This is the **character ethic**. You have the time to foster relationships and you will (7 Habits of Highly Effective People). When you see patients in the inpatient setting you aren't afforded the time to build that kind of relationship. But it's just as necessary that they trust, like, and connect with you. Instead, you must employ the **personality ethic** (How to Win Friends and Influence People). Yes, on some level that means manipulating people. Don't freak out. Remember, you're in the business of helping people. Sometimes you just need to help them let you help them.

1. **Bedside rounds:** Do it with your attending or resident. When patients see how much intellectual energy goes into their care they'll be amazed. Rather than discussing the case in the HIPAA-non-compliant hallway followed by the 30 second drive-by conversation in the room, try having the entire patient discussion in the room. Yes, they'll interrupt. Yep, they'll ask questions. And sure, this isn't ALWAYS appropriate, but most of the time it is. Show them how much time you spend on them.

2. **Sit down:** When you sit in a patient's room, whether on a chair, the bed, or just kneeling nearby, patients think you're in the room twice as long as you are. Standing relays a mental cue of you wanting to leave, which results in patients rating you as being in the room half as long as you are. So sit down (that said, stand if your attending is in the room and standing - don't look lazy or uncaring).

3. **Uncross your arms and face the patient:** Use open body language at all times. Lean in towards them. Keep your hands at your side or in front of you gesturing. Point with an open palm, not with a finger. Turn your body (not just your head) towards your patient. Open body language is a surefire way to gain some trust and subconscious person points.

4. **Use Names:** The most important word to any person is their own name. Ask how the patient wishes to be referred to. Remember it and use it. "Mr. Dustyn, Mr. Williams, Dustyn, Captain Cheesecake McBurgerberry." If they make a joke name, use it with a smile. If they share a name of their child, spouse, or anyone else, write it down in your data tracker. It has meaning to the patient, thus it has utility for you. Use these names the next time you see them. Oh yeah... and TELL THEM YOURS.

PATIENT SATISFACTION

5. **Touch people:** I don't mean do a physical (you're going to do that always anyway). I mean touch people: their hand if they're upset, their leg if discussing a relevant diagnosis there etc. Of course there's too much touching. There's inappropriate touching too. If I have to spell it out we're in trouble and you should stop reading now. But offer a handshake. It's OK to hug a patient or a family member (don't do this a lot). It's MORE than OK to comfort someone with the power of touch.

6. **Smile:** Sincerely. Unless it's a somber event or bad news, smile. People like smiling.

7. **Treat people like people, not like patients or diseases:** Patients are people first. Treat them with the same respect and diligence you would any human being. You're not a robot and they're not a stone. Connect emotionally and you'll win the hearts and trust of your patients. This one is vague, and likely an advanced skill for many, but also what will ultimately fend off your replacement, IBM Watson. This also means getting away from your COW or computer terminal and to the bedside.

8. **Give them choices:** Lights on or off, covers up or down, head of the bed up or down, TV on or off, blinds opened or closed. They're in the hospital; they can do NOTHING for themselves. Medications come at the whim of the EMR and the nurse. Meals come when dietary brings it (unless your nurse is awesome and will get them a snack when they want it). Patients are NPO (eating really matters to patients). They're woken up every 2 hours all day long. They have NO CONTROL. Allow them to get some back by offering choices when possible. No matter how small, tell them, through your actions "I get it, this situation sucks, but I see you as a person and not a pin cushion for me to draw labs from."

9. **Don't fret:** You're going to mess up or say things they might not like to hear. There will be a patient that doesn't want to see you anymore. They want the, "real doctor." Do two things. First, reflect: did you do something to cause this? Second, comply: let it roll off your shoulders - some people are just that way. Don't get caught up, but don't ignore it either. Chances are it's a learning moment for you.

10. **Disney World:** You buy a T-shirt at Disney World on Day 1 of a 14 day trip. You destroy it: use, abuse, stain it, and rip off the sleeves. On the way out of the park on day 14, if you ask to exchange it for a brand new one and Disney will do it. A brand new shirt even though you ruined your first one. Know why? No matter how amazing the experience was for those 14 days, if you leave with a, "man, they're so stingy, it's just a shirt," mentality it will be the lasting memory that sticks. Regardless of how good the experience, when patients prepare to leave the hospital, spend time with them and give them their T-shirt. A few narcotics, a phone call to their son who is in medical school, a refill on a medication they don't NEED from you, a work excuse - these things go a LONG way and cost you nothing.

25

Survival Techniques

Life is hard.

Residency is harder.

Good News.

You aren't the first to go through it.

You won't be the last.

Learn from those before you. Heed their teachings; take advantage of their success and their failure.

"To have striven, to have made the effort, to have been true to certain ideals – this alone is worth the struggle. "
– *Sir William Osler*

CHAPTER 2: SURVIVAL TECHNIQUES

Time Management: Data Tracking

The Data Tracker is a means of taking every new patient from the ED to discharge. It makes daily rounding super easy. It lets H&Ps and Discharge Summaries flow. No more clicking through 15 tabs while sitting there on the phone all confused. Move on from empty Epic templates with meaningless information that no one wants or cares to see. Look like AND know what you're doing.

Find ours on the resources tab of the dashboard at onlinemeded.org (free, just register).

Types of Data

There are two things you want on your data tracker: the static and the daily.

The **static data** is the information that won't change. Some of it should be obvious (name, date of birth, MRN, acct number, PmHx, PsHx, Soc Hx, All, FamHx, Home Meds), but some may not. The major categories in the H&P form should go in the static data. But you also want to include the big tests: major diagnostics, procedures, and past information. That's going to change depending said diagnosis. This is where **culture data, CT scans / MRIs**, echo results, cath results, etc. are going to go. It's NOT part of the daily data (it will be for one day) but you want it easily accessible at all times. You put the **surgeries** and procedures here too. Finally, the **day of presentation** goes in the static data (the vitals, labs, and pertinent physical exam). This static data is the important info for the **H&P** and **Discharge Summary**.

The **daily data** are the points you want to track: vitals, labs, meds etc. You want to be able to track trends. It'll let you see what happened day to day, better or worse. This is where you're going to **present from daily**. Literally. On rounds, you will tell your story; you know what the subjective and what the plan is... but how do you remember all those labs and vitals? You don't. Since you know the gist of what's going on, you tell the story, then you look down at this tracker and read off the details, then continue the story. This is just to have the details written down to refer to later.

Whatever you choose, ideally **static data** is on **one side** while **daily data is on the other**. An example, "the notecard" is shown on the next page.

For meds you best get yourself a **pencil**. They change all the time. Every day you're going to sit in front of a computer. Every day you will run through the meds. Whatever you pick (I always liked separating scheduled from prn) the meds will be displayed in the same order every day. You just quickly go through and mark changes. And because medications change daily, you will either want to leave space and/or be able to erase meds or dosages.

Time Management: Data Tracking

Front of Card (Admit Day)

Dustyn Williams
10/23/1951
64 yo m Chest Pain

Acct: 1005123678
MRN: 0025816
Admit: 256184 | 3/5
Disch:

PMHx	PSHx	Meds	All	SocHx
HTN	2 Stents	ASA 81	NKDA	1. Tob: 30py quit '08
DM	Lap Chole	Plavix 75		2. EtOH ∅
└Retin	Appy	Metop 50"	FamHx	3. Drugs ∅
└Neuro		Lisinp 40	♀: CVA	4. Lives: wife
└Nephr		Atorva 80	♂: MI	⊕ADLs
CAD		Metformin 500"		5. PCP:
HLD				Roge Borgia
CHD II				

5' 11"   195 lbs

160/100   120   24   98⁷   100%

⊕Neuropathy   Non pleuritic
Cool feet   Non positional
∅Bruit   Non tender
∅murmur

9.6 ⤬ 15 / 394

142 | 106 | 0.9 ⟋ 98
3.7 | 24 | 18

Old ♡:
1. LHC '09   90% OM₁ (Stent)
2. LHC '13   90% OM₂ (Stent)
   40% RCA (∅stent)
3. Echo '14   EF 55%
   PAP 45

ECG: Old Infarct
CXR: ⊖
Troponin: 0.01
            0.02

Stress:

Back of Card (Daily)

ASA 81	98⁷ 64-84 12-16 142-160/88 - 100		1. CAD
Atorva 80	8 ⤬ 15/342 140 | 116 | 1.0 ⟋ 97		└ LHC
Plavix 75	(3.7) | 24 | 0.9		└ CABG
	∅SSI needed ⊕Stress		
Lovenox 40	99' 66-72 12-14 123-142/66-88		2. DM
Lisinopril 40	142 | 116 | 12 ⟋ 102		3. HTN
metoprolol 50"/100	4.2 | 24 | 1.1		4. HLD
	∅SSI. Cath → Multivessel Disease		5. Out PPx
Lantus 10	102' 108-122 24-36 (T) MAP: 84-92		6. Dispo
+SSI qAc	16 ⤬ 10/182 (156) | 122 | 36' ⟋ 98		
	(3.2) | 30 | 1.1		
	NG Tube Central Line		
	ET Tube Foley		

CHAPTER 2:   SURVIVAL TECHNIQUES

Some options:

1. **Note Cards –**   *Your iPad and the*
   a.   PROS   *COW don't count!*
      i.   Toss them when the patient discharges.
      ii. Can easily expand another card for patients with long stays.
   b.   CONS
      i.   Losable. If you hole-punch a corner and keep them on a ring, you can avoid this lose-ability potential, but finding the right patient can become a challenge unless you maintain organization (ie every day by room).
      ii. Less space than a book to keep data.
2. **The Book –**
   a.   PROS
      i.   Really hard to lose. If you lose it, generally it finds its ways back.
      ii. Never falls apart; can be kept forever.
   b.   CONS
      i.   Heavy. It might weigh down your white coat.
      ii. If a patient stays for a long time there may not be enough space and it's hard to go back and forth to your current position and to that patient's.

Use Shorthand – These are your notes in your tracker so efficiency > beauty. Use hash marks for the number of times a day a medication is given, the sticks for CBC, BMP, LFT, and write annotated reports from the scans.

Wait - this sounds like a lot of work. Why should I do it?

Does filling out a data tracker **take more time**? Yes. On the day of admit it takes more time. Is it **less convenient** than just printing out your autopopulated note for the day? Yes. So why would you tell me to do this?

1. **Let it be your written H&P.** Your dictated H&P and oral presentation will be flawless if you use this. Also, there's no need to write out a beautiful hand-written H&P AND dictate.
2. **Let it be your written Discharge summary.** Here is where it saves time. All the data is in front of you. There's no fight for a computer terminal; you don't have to flip back and forth between tabs, watching the spinning wheel of death tell you "loading…".
3. **You know your patients better.** Residency is about training. The data tracker will force you to engage vitals, labs, and meds. They won't have been recorded simply for the sake of it. You'll have seen and thought about them, which will better prepare you for rounds. Trends will be easier to detect. When stressed by heavy throughput you WON'T MISS ANYTHING because you developed the mental discipline to use this tracker.

You're going to end up needing this information anyway (rounds, H&P, D/C).
You're going to write this information down every day anyway.
It might as well be in an efficient format.

Time Management: To Do Lists / Scut Lists

The To-Do list is a crucial component of your day to day work. It has nothing to do with making you better as a doctor or learning anything. It does, however, **manage your sanity** and prevent orders from falling through the cracks. It helps ensure no patients get hurt, but really it's about you. Here are some things the To-Do list should be:

Transportable. The To-Do list should easily fit in a white coat pocket or any other means that lends itself to portability.

Paper.

You want to be able to see it all at a glance. Like, all of it. Being on a cell phone or an iPad won't do. You won't be able to see how much there's to be done or easily make small adjustments. Being able to write things down, to have the paper conform to your needs rather than your texts conform to the rules of the device, is crucial. If you're really slick (and don't mind carrying different colored pens), color coding is helpful.

Disposable.

You want to be able to throw away your To-Do list at the end of the day. Once everything is complete, it's satisfying to discard it (in a designated shred box to prevent HIPAA issues). It also represents finality to your day; "I can go home now." It's definitely a positive charge to emotional battery pack (see emotional bank account). Disposable doesn't mean "push the trash icon." Make it paper; I promise it'll be better. Just be certain not to lose it.

Separate from your data tracking method.

While it'd be nice to double your data tracking method with your to-do list, it'll inevitably make your data tracker messy. Likewise, it's a daily to-do list – there's no need to remind yourself of all the work that had to get done yesterday. Most of the points on the list are just tasks you don't want to carry around throughout the hospitalization.

How I (Dustyn) did mine:
Take an 8.5 x 11 piece of a paper and fold it in half so that you still have an 11" sheet. Then fold it again once in the opposite axis. Continue to do so until you have enough rectangles for all your patients. If you fold once, you get 4 rectangles. Fold again to get 8 rectangles, one more time for 16 rectangles. 8 is ideal for the intern, while 16 is ideal for the resident.

This isn't a place to put labs and vitals. This isn't a tracker. Just put a checkbox next to a task for that patient and check as you complete the task.

I can't overemphasize developing this skill early in your career. It's immediately translatable to work as an upper level resident (where you have to manage twice as many patients and two subordinate interns). It also can be translated to staff work as an attending. Here are some examples: Intern, Resident, then Attending. The details aren't important - just see how many iterations of this same process there are and how useful they can be.

CHAPTER 2:   SURVIVAL TECHNIQUES

All patient information shown is fabricated. The intern (left) has just their information. The resident (below) has the to-do list separated by intern, which allows them to use it to guide the team room to room. It also lets them "run the list" with each intern to ensure that all tasks for the day have been recorded or done. The resident can then offer autonomy to the interns and check back later in the day marking off tasks as they are completed (now able to check them off remotely).

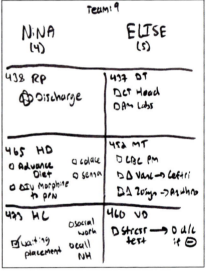

The attending view demos how they can mark down what they need to do in regards to billing or attestations. They can also take on the role of the resident listed above. Note that attending + resident scuts are only half the sheet - we showed enough to get the gist and bolded it so you can actually read it.

TIME MANAGEMENT: TO DO LISTS / SCUT LISTS

Mastering Time Management As you begin putting this together you'll see how one piece of time saving merges with another. When you identify **Turkeys and Windows** (See that section in Time Management) and learn how to prioritize **important and urgent** tasks (see that section in Time Management) you'll see how fluid your life can be. It should also help visualize how UN-daunting your to-do list is.

When starting, it'll be tempting to check off a bunch of really easy and insignificant tasks just to make the list look like it's not so big (look how much you've accomplished!). That's ok; there's a sense of reward or accomplishment that comes with checking those boxes. You'll also need those positive motivators.

But soon you'll get into the habit of recognizing what does and doesn't need to be finished right now. You won't be plagued by a long list because you'll know it's full of things that are easy to do and can be done later. Instead, your focus will turn to the things that really NEED to be done immediately. Days will become much more efficient than you realized possible.

SURVIVAL

CHAPTER 2: SURVIVAL TECHNIQUES

Survival Skills: Morning Workflow

Before the Upper Level Resident /Attending – early morning flow

1. The computer / data mining
All data is in the computer nowadays. It's essential to go through that information before your day gets going.

Sit down at a computer. Pull out your **data tracker**. Go through and copy down **vitals** and **labs**. Review the **medications**. Take notes on **imaging, subspecialist input**, and ancillary recommendations (**PT, OT**).

For your 5-7 patients this should take 15-20 minutes.

Based on **vitals, labs**, and **nursing reports** you should be able to identify the 3 Ds, which are **Death** (1st), **Discharge** (2nd), and **Diagnosis** (3rd). This prioritizes who you see and in which order. Don't save the ICU for the end – they're the most ill.

2. The patients
See your patients. **As an intern, the goal is to get information**. How'd they do overnight, are there any new complaints? As bravery builds (second half of the year), you can start talking about what you plan on doing.

While you should follow the 3Ds, let's be realistic. You're likely going to see everyone in a geographic location first as it saves on time back and forth. So plan your route before standing and leaving the computer.

It's a good idea to see the talkative ones early. You can always use the line, "alright, I have other patients to check on. We'll come back and we can keep talking then" (because you're coming back on rounds). If you do this, **you must come back** that day. Cha-ching, easy deposit.

3. The notes
Back to the **computer** you go. Try to get notes done before resident rounds. Use your Data Tracker and Rounds on patients. If you can't get it finished, that's ok. It's more important to have your plan ready and orders in the system than to have your notes done for rounds.

DO use copy and paste from previous notes
DO make sure you aren't wastefully copying over nonsense.

Update:
1. Vitals
2. Labs
3. Meds
4. Assessment and Plan

Survival Skills: Morning Workflow

It's an awesome time saver to let autopopulating notes just autopopulate. They look stupid, which makes you look stupid. But it's ok to do it, because it does save time. Still, do this sparingly. Make your stuff look good. For billing, for communication. Make it look like you actually wrote it and didn't let a computer write it for you.

SAMPLE DAY

<u>6:30am</u> arrive at the hospital and sit down at a computer terminal. Fill out data tracker.

<u>7:00am</u> morning report.

<u>8:00am</u> *see patients.*
- <u>D</u>ying: barring a crashing patient or someone you identified to be in trouble based on labs and vitals, you should be able to round freely and geographically. It's about obtaining information at this point. If someone is in trouble, call your upper level immediately.

<u>9:00am</u> *the "other D's"*
- <u>D</u>iagnosis: put in orders NOW... aka early. Get ahead of the other resident teams who will wait until after attending rounds to put their orders in.
- <u>D</u>ischarge: inform social workers, nurses, and patient families that the person might go home. If the plan yesterday was to discharge them today, activate that discharge.
- <u>D</u>iscuss: talk to your upper level resident about the plan for the day. Make sure you're ready for rounds and that a plan has been developed AND enacted.

<u>10:00am</u> *Attending Rounds*
- The attending comes through and sees patients with you.
- Coaching happens.
- Plans are critiqued and uncertainties are laid to rest.

<u>12:00pm</u> *Work Time*
- Do what came up on Attending Rounds.
- Save lunch for when the lines are short and the space abundant (go at 1, not 12).

<u>1:00 – 3:00pm</u> *Procedures and Meetings*
- Set family discussions, paracenteses, thoracenteses, etc. for this time block.
- Use this time to start writing notes if there's nothing else to do.

<u>3:00pm – 5:00pm</u> *Notes and New Patients*
- Finish your notes by 4:00pm. The To-Do list should be mostly checked off.
- If you're on Short or Long call, here's where you'll start to pick up new patients from the ED. This time (1:00 – 5:00) can be sort of a jumble, depending on when patients come in.

<u>5:00pm – 7:00pm</u> Go home or finish off your call.

CHAPTER 2:   SURVIVAL TECHNIQUES

Survival Skills: Urgent and Important

Urgent and Important: deciding what to do first

Other people define urgency. Everyone thinks what they need to get done is most important. And to them it might be; their to-do list is different from yours. Indeed, maybe that case manager getting the order to change to inpatient truly has nothing more important to do than that. But because other people define those tasks, they'll pressure you to get them done. And you'll want to do them, even if they have no utility for your day.

You define importance, and in the case of hospital wards, the things that **get your patients what they need are important** (this is different than importance in the relevance vs importance argument for clinical reasoning). Stay focused on important tasks; don't be distracted by urgent ones. As long as your focus is patient care - getting your patients what they need - you'll always be in the right.

Those tasks which are **both urgent and important** always go first (rapid response is a great example). From there the waterfall is important tasks, urgent tasks, then just tasks.

URGENT

		YES	NO
IMPORTANT	YES	** First **	Second
	NO	Third	Last

Of course, there are exceptions. For example, multidisciplinary rounds are a time where case managers, social workers, and nursing staff come together to get stuff done. Some of that might be NOT important and NOT urgent. But since it's the designated time to do it you'd do those tasks at that time.

Prioritizing tasks will make your life immensely more effective.

SURVIVAL SKILLS: URGENT AND IMPORTANT

Saying no, and telling people they have to wait

When someone comes at you with an urgent task (urgent for you, important to them) you have to be able to say no. But saying, "That isn't important, I'll do it later," will compromise the emotional bank account, zap the emotional battery, and shatter relationships. Soon enough, you'll be called into the program director's office and blame all your troubles on RBF (if you don't know what this is you probably don't have it, but urban dictionary it anyway).

You want to show them you care, but also not get distracted from more important tasks.

The key here is to make people **feel they've been heard and that you get them**. Providing specific reasons why you can't do their task right now is a great approach. "I can't come down to fill out that paper med rec just yet. I'm in the ED with a patient right now. As soon as I'm done with this admit I'll come up." Another way is to show them your list. Write down their task on your scut-list / to-do list. **Let them see you write it**. If they can't, tell them it's been written down. They'll have the comfort of knowing it's been taken off their plate and added to yours.

Defining the Important Tasks, the 3 D's

Death, **D**iagnosis, **D**ischarge. Anything that has to do with the 3 D's goes to the top of the list. If the task doesn't, it goes to the bottom. This includes paperwork and notes.

Remember that some tasks have a wait time (they're your Turkeys). Get ahead of the line by ordering them first. But in general, what you want to do is this:

1. **Diagnostic tests** – get ahead of the line by putting these orders or making the call early.
2. **Consults** – get the calls in early, else you may delay the consultant to the next day.
3. **Discharge** – the point of 1 and 2 is to get the patient ready for discharge the day BEFORE they go home. Those you know are ready to go home today get that process started as early as possible.
4. **Orders** – this is self-explanatory. Anything left over that needs to be done that won't immediately get the patient discharged (#3) or closer to discharge (Turkeys: #1, #2) is done next.
5. **Procedures** – Assure you leave enough time before and after the procedure to get it done. This sounds like #1, but when YOU have to do the procedure you don't want to be rushed for time, else you might make a mistake.
6. **Family Conferences** – schedule these at the end of the day.
7. **Daily Notes** – these don't need to be ready for rounds. You have your data tracker and know what's going on. You put in orders already (#4). Don't let yourself get time-crunched by the start of rounds. Know what's going on. Do prepare for your patients. Document it later.   Since you'll have more results and information from the day, your notes (and sign out) will be better.

CHAPTER 2: SURVIVAL TECHNIQUES

Time Management: Turkeys and Windows

The wards are a challenging place with many moving parts. The day can be broken into snippets of time (pre-rounds, morning report, resident rounds, attending rounds, work rounds). It's comfortable to give each of these time periods their own tasks. That is, *"I'll wait to put in the orders after attending rounds during work rounds, because that's where order-entry belongs."* This is folly for many reasons and your efficiency will be grossly compromised unless you understand Turkeys and Windows.

Turkeys

In the mind of the intern you enter an order and that order happens. Presto, chango, donezo. What many young physicians don't realize are the chain of events that must occur before the action actually happens. It involves a many people. People hold things up.

Let's use the blood draw as an example.

For you: I want a CBC. <Click CBC>. Why isn't the CBC back yet?

Reality: You want a CBC. You log into the EMR and order it. The lab receives the order and assigns a number to it. That order is transmitted to the nursing staff, which acknowledges it. If it's a STAT or NURSE DRAW order, the nurse will do this next part. If it's not, the phlebotomist is dispatched to collect the lab. They arrive in the room with a cart, wrap that blue elastic band around the patient's arm, look for a place to stick, do so and draw the blood. The lab slip is affixed to the vial and it's either sent or brought to the lab. The lab tech processes the blood, but most likely in a batch of 30 other vials. The computer reports a value and the lab tech enters that data into the computer system. Your EMR flags the patient as having a new lab value and you see the lab.
Feel the difference?

Every lab you order means the patient will get stuck with a needle. Batch them. If anyone in the chain has something more important to do your order gets delayed. If other people have orders in ahead of yours, you'll go to the back of the line and have yours processed in sequence.

So what's with the Turkey? If you've ever prepared Thanksgiving dinner you know it centers around that Turkey. The Turkey is big; it takes up the entire oven. It also needs to be cooked for like... 12 hours. Other foods need to be prepared too, but the Turkey has to be started the day before to make it ready for dinner. If you begin cooking a 16 pound bird two hours before dinner, it won't be ready and everyone will get salmonella. Everything needs to be cooked and ready at 3pm for dinner, but due to space limitations it can't all be done at once. Therefore, it's essential to **plan the cooking appropriately**; things that **need more time get started earlier.**

The best example I can think of is an MRI. The MRI is the turkey. If you wait until noon (work rounds) to order the MRI you'll be competing with every other team who wants

38

Time Management: Turkeys and Windows

one. There's only one MRI machine and it can hold exactly one patient at a time. Most MRI procedures take more than an hour. Then it must be read. So treat it like a turkey - start your MRI early. You can work on the discharges of other patients while waiting for the MRI results to come back. Then, by 3pm, "dinner is ready," and you're out of here. Compare this to waiting until noon, where you likely won't have the result until well after you've left, which means it's tabled, "for tomorrow."

Windows
The day is divided into time-slots, which are windows. I've alluded to windows already in Turkeys. Things that need more time need to get started earlier. You have **windows of opportunity** to get things done. If you miss them they're gone.

Most teams will wait until after rounds to actually do things. You've probably already been there as a medical student. At 1:30pm no one has eaten lunch; the residents are all furiously putting in orders, calling consults, and finishing notes. You stood there asking, "Is there anything I can do to help," which really meant, "I'm hungry, can I please go eat lunch?" It probably seemed like the right thing. This was work-time and the residents were working.

But what if you, now the resident and no longer the student, used windows of opportunities to make your day more efficient? You know the social worker will need to know that this person is going home later today. So tell her. You know this person will need a CT scan. Order it. The point is **you have to know when to do something**. This is different than the 3Ds (dying, discharge, diagnosis). It's an extra layer of complexity and must be in the context of your day and the patient census.

Specifically, you don't want to just check the boxes on your to-do list. You need to **prioritize tasks, recognize how long each will take to accomplish, when they need to be started**, and how **much time will have to be committed to it**. Once the process is started, unless YOU'RE doing the task (like a thoracentesis) you're freed to do something else.

Consider this example: You know interventional radiology doesn't work after 3pm, the patient hasn't gotten lovenox yet today, and will likely need a lumbar puncture that you won't be able to perform on your own (due to bad anatomy). What do you do? Be honest with yourself. Right now you would write a note saying, "consult IR today," then wait until after rounds to put in the call. The patient will have gotten lovenox and the IR LP will get done tomorrow. ORRRRRRRRRRRRR, you could hold the lovenox, call IR, get the LP done, and later write your note with included CSF results from the procedure that happened today. Plus, while that LP is happening you also discharge three other patients and order the CT scan for patient number 5.

Lessons learned:
1. Things that take more time should be started earlier
2. Limited resources should be utilized when no one else has thought to use them
3. Make decisions. Come to rounds ready to say what you did rather than ask what you should do

CHAPTER 2: SURVIVAL TECHNIQUES

People Management: Relationships

Relationships with others: The Bank Account

Every relationship is like a checking account; there are **deposits** and **withdrawals**. When you've been friends with someone for a long time there have been many deposits made, a withdrawal can be made without hurting the relationship. When the relationship is new (you just met the nurse on the floor for the first time), and no deposits have been made, small withdrawals can overdraw the account.

Translate this to friendship. Your long-time friend comes into town to visit. You have a lunch date scheduled but their meeting runs late. They text saying they can't make it and they'll meet up with you at the end of your shift for drinks. You say ok.

Now you've recently started residency and want to make some friends. You're supposed to meet one of the ER residents for happy hour on Friday afternoon, but you're running late on an extra discharge. The anxiety you feel about being late is appropriate as you don't want to make a bad impression. Worse, if you stand them up you may not have another opportunity. Same goes for when the boss asks you to a football game. You don't decline - you obsess over the clothes you'll wear and are sure to arrive early.

Every relationship has a bank account. The goal is to **add deposits whenever possible**. Deposits strengthen a relationship. The more deposits and the more trust, the more likely that person is willing to do for you what they won't for others. **People are people.** No matter how good someone is at their job or how much they care, if they don't like you it's inevitable that you'll get less from them. Whether nurses will have the ultrasound in the room, consent signed, and all equipment ready before you arrive isn't a product of their dedication to the job, but rather their dedication to you. They could've just as easily gotten the central line kit from central and left you to get consent and the ultrasound yourself.

How do you add deposits? Deposits are **NOT favors**. In reality you can do very little for the clerk, the nurse, or the unit manager. You write notes and orders. Instead, what you can do is **listen** and **show genuine interest in people**. Listen to how that 5 center nurse talks about her 4 kids and her stay-at-home-dad-husband. That 3 north nurse likes to drink beer, heard that you had a Kegerator installed, and spent 15 minutes talking about what beer you should get next. The social worker is pregnant, but she's only 14 weeks and doesn't show yet. **Listen** to what they talk about, **talk to them** about those things, and **use their name**. When you make a commitment, a promise, **follow through on that commitment**. If you fail them, **apologize sincerely**.

This chit-chat may seem like a waste of time; it's probably getting in their way and slowing them down. You actually don't care - you just want them to do their job. Why do you have to motivate them to do what you ask? Well, because they're human beings and that's how human beings work.

40

PEOPLE MANAGEMENT: RELATIONSHIPS

DON'T get in their way. But when there's downtime build that relationship with people on the team. Like a bank account, I assure you it'll pay off with interest in the end.

Discharge	Recharge	Withdrawal	Deposit
Exhaustion	Sleep	Lying	Truthfulness
Isolation	Friends	Not showing up	Keeping commitments
Reprimand	Praise	Hearing	Listening
Loss	Hobbies	Talking	Paying Attention
Life in the hospital	Life outside medicine	Ignoring people	Attending the details
Satisfying others needs	Meeting your own needs	Charlatan	Sincerity
		Blame	Apologies

Relationships with self: The Emotional Battery

People are people. No matter how much you think of yourself, you're a person too. You aren't immortal or invincible. You need sleep and praise (or at least acknowledgement).

Here's the thing. When coming back from a week-long vacation where all you did was get drunk and sit on the beach, your emotional battery is fully charged. Someone cracks a sarcastic joke about your shoes; no worries, it rolls right off your shoulders. The battery gets drained a little, but whatever, it's still at 98%. At 98% charge your phone is still on max brightness, full color, and you're surfing Facebook instead of writing notes.

Then the wards start. 1 day off in 7. 80 hours a week. Just through work, people make withdrawals from your bank account. This is ok, because when people make a withdrawal you're depositing into their account. But every withdrawal drains your emotional battery a little bit. Then you have a rough call day. You don't sleep well for two days in a row. Suddenly, you're at 10%. Like your phone on a call day ("BOOP BOOP battery low"), if you're at 10% on hour 6 of 16, you turn your brightness down, turn on power saving mode, and stop playing Clash of Clans.

Now you reach into your bag for the charger. Whoops, left it at home. What happens? You panic; you NEED your phone. Even more so on call day. Now anxiety is going up. The frantic low battery texts go out; you start asking for a charger from everyone you know.

41

CHAPTER 2: SURVIVAL TECHNIQUES

When your emotional battery gets critically low the withdrawals matter more. The blood starts to boil and you have vicious outbursts. You become more emotionally labile and now you're crying. Wait, how did we arrive here?

There are two dangers to this scenario:

The first is what a **low battery does to others**. Your disproportionate reactions to people will cause massive withdrawals from emotional bank accounts. Your reactions will be disproportionate to the stressor. You lose your filter (power-save mode) and all the energy it takes to be polite in society won't be there. You know how to act (your forebrain) but you'll react (your amygdala). The midbrain will win.

The second is what a **low battery does to you**. This is how anger and depression creep in (Death and Dying in Residency). They don't happen all at once, but operating at a critically low power level for too long, or worse, draining to power off will push you into these bad stages of death and dying in residency. Think of this to help you understand why someone has a bad reaction, an outburst, or a crying spell to something you think is innocuous. It isn't that they're weak, it's that they're drained.

You need time to recharge. You also have to find out what constitutes a recharge. If that's talking to your significant other on the phone, then do it. Just make sure your partner isn't critically low or that talking to you isn't a deposit into your account from their battery (what recharges you may drain others). You want to find things that recharge you and don't drain others. Just remember that those things (even sleeping) can be either a deposit or withdrawal from someone else. With the complexities and stresses of ward life, most people are probably operating near 20% charge.

To stay off the battery low message, you have to know yourself. Pay attention to the small things. Treat yourself. Have a nice meal, go to the park, get to the gym, spend time with your kids. Whatever it is for you, you have to keep it up. The mental, emotional, and time commitment you devote during residency is costly. There won't be enough time to keep up with every hobby and friend. SO.... What you do needs to count.

Surround yourself with people who make you better. Learn to say no to relationships that drain you and benefit you little. You don't need new friends (unless you do). Rely on those with whom you've built a strong relationship with. Keep a hobby. Do something you enjoy. Sleep.

You want to make deposits into others' bank account. You must recharge your battery. Residency is hard. It can be harder if you fail to cultivate strong relationships. It's hardest if you try to function with a depleted battery.

42

PEOPLE MANAGEMENT: BEING EFFECTIVE

People Management: Being Effective

This ISN'T about right and wrong. Nor is it about what you should or shouldn't do. This is about being effective. Specifically, **being effective** for your patient. You must walk into the wards with the perspective of, "*everything I'm going to do today is to help my patients.*" That's why you're in medicine. You might THINK that everyone else will have the same motivation - they won't. To be effective for your patient you'll have to get people to do what you want them to do. As long as you use your powers for good (helping the patient), you can take solace in the fact that **you'll be manipulating people**.

Manipulation carries a negative connotation, but it shouldn't. It's the same thing as motivation. It's also the same thing as management. Here, it's about getting people's goals aligned so that, as a team, we can be effective in delivering patient care.

Remember that everything you ask someone to do is a withdrawal from their emotional bank account. Every time you put in an order, make a change, or request something it drains both the person and your relationship with them a little bit. Most of what you ask for are within the job description, so it won't cause that much of a withdrawal. But, remember that 1) people are people and 2) most people on the wards are operating around a 20% charge.

Thus, when **you want someone to do something** it's imperative to **make that withdrawal as small as possible** and figure out how **your request aligns with their goals**.

This is why you spend so much time depositing into the emotional bank account. Not only does it build trust with the person you deposit into, you also learn what makes them tick. **Listening and really caring about other people** is how relationships are forged. Sometimes, your relationship will be so strong, the trust in you so high, that the person will help simply because you asked, which is enough. This is the benefit of **unit-based rounding** where physicians join nursing teams rather than floating between floors.

However, most of the time you won't have a terrific relationship to fall on. Your reputation will NOT likely precede you. As such, you'll have to convince the person that what you're asking is reasonable and should be done. Do it by using what you know about them from all that time you've spent building up the bank account.

It likely won't be done with a logical argument; it's hard to explain the necessity of why to someone with little knowledge of the patient and/or medicine. You have to make them **feel it**.

You have 17 things to do, one of which is to complete this task. You have your reasons. The person you need to do it also has 17 things to do, one of which is also to get this done. They also have their reasons to get other tasks done. The key is to increase your task's priority by aligning **why** it should be done with their own values. No one's values are better than another's – they're just different. They have to be aligned in order to make anything happen.

43

CHAPTER 2: SURVIVAL TECHNIQUES

People Management: Arguments

Arguments are going to happen. Remember, your job is to be **effective** - not right or wrong. Effective means "doing good for your patient." If you can do that well, so much the better.

First Rule of arguments: you're both wrong. If one person was obviously correct, there would be no argument. The gunshot victim with 14 holes in his abdomen is going to surgery, the 22-year-old without vital sign abnormality or laboratory change is going home. But that's not where fights happen. They happen over ambiguity. Your job is to find out where you're wrong or where a miscommunication has happened.

Second rule of arguments: emotion always loses. "I think" and "I feel" go up against "you said" and "you think." Clash. And not "of clans." In this kind of fight the person with the loudest, strongest emotion will win. If you're lucky enough to be the louder person, congrats (see rule #3). If you're unlucky, you'll have this emotional outburst fight in front of others. Withdrawals all around. Everyone who sees you get emotional will immediately have massive withdrawals from their emotional bank account. You aren't supposed to be a machine (letting off steam, commiserating with staff, high-fiving the nurses are all ok). But, doing so in an argument - no. Here's the thing; the person you're arguing with is emotionally attached to their position. Their position is them. Same for you – you are your position. In this scenario, neither person can surrender, else they surrender themselves.

Instead, search for the third alternative - the solution is something neither of you saw perfectly. To do that you should focus on **facts**. Maybe the surgery resident hasn't seen the CT scan that you have. Maybe you need to examine the patient together; three hours ago they weren't peritoneal, but now they are. **Facts**, not emotions, are going to make you **effective**. More importantly, it's likely the patient will win (and so will you and the arguer).

Third rule of arguments: when you win, you lose. Effectiveness, relationships, emotional bank accounts, batteries; these are all getting dinged if it's an outright win for you. This can be true even if the first two rules of arguments are met. You think the person in a persistent vegetative state needs a PEG tube, because that's your value. Three GI attendings say no since they know it's futile. You continue arguing with the third and eventually the patient gets a PEG tube. You won! But now you've marked yourself as a problem, a wacko, or worse. You've also compromised the relationship with the fellow by twisting their arm to do what you wanted.

Forth rule of arguments: get help. If the **third alternative** can't be reached, step back. This is the benefit of being in training. There's always someone to fall back on. You **shouldn't be a doormat**; don't get stepped on or overlooked. You **shouldn't be a pest**; don't get a reputation as the person who tries to push other people around. You **don't want to be a snitch**; don't run behind people all the time. BUT, if a resolution can't be reached, **CALL YOUR ATTENDING.** For whatever reason, attendings are much cooler

PEOPLE MANAGEMENT: ARGUMENTS

with each other than residents are with each other. We fight A LOT less. If you're in trouble or think patient care is getting compromised, call your attending. Staff to staff conversations happen all the time. The egos are larger, but there's less to prove and more to lose if a patient (or a relationship) gets compromised.

Top 10 Practical Pointers For Winning Arguments.

1. Talk in a soft, monotone voice. Don't show emotion. You're about facts. No condescension, sarcasm, or patronizing.
2. Stand with your arms straight and at your sides. Gesturing is threatening (non-verbal emotion) and crossing your arms is condescending. The person will hear your body language much louder than your words
3. Listen
4. Listen
5. Listen
6. Listen. I don't mean hear or anticipate what you're going to say next. Debates are about retorting and twisting the person's words back against them. Don't Debate. In an argument about a patient, accept that what the person is saying is correct, or, at least that their opinion matters. Maybe you're wrong. At the very least, since there's an argument in the first place, your information is likely incomplete. Figure out where by listening.
7. Admit it when you're wrong. Say the words "the truth matters to me more than being right or wrong, I want what is best for the patient".
8. Agree first. Find out where the two of you align. Say what you agree on. Use it to build the case. You're going to have your chance to talk. When you do, get to the point. Agree on point 1, 2, and 3. But wait - here is where we disagree. Shift away from "you, me" and towards "us, we" – that's the third alternative.
9. Give them a way out. You've listened and see where the facts went awry. He can't separate himself or his ego from the argument. Do that for him. Point to a FACT that he either didn't know, hadn't considered, or misinterpreted. His value and opinion can change with this new consideration. You and I know the CT scan was there all along, but use it to help him to separate his ego from the argument.
10. **If all else fails, lose the fight**. You know about this emotional burden, this issue of ego. The person you're arguing with doesn't. Thus, you won't see it as loss or be drained by it. Give them a win; you just deposited into their bank account. At the very least, you didn't make a withdrawal. Then, knowing you're right, employ rule # 4 and you call your attending. Staff to staff. You win, twice.

chapter 2: Survival Techniques

Life Management: In Your Box

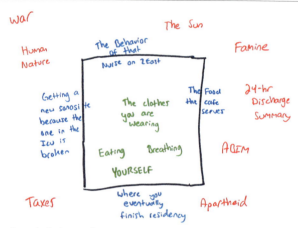

Ask the question: is it in my box? Is it in my sphere of influence?
There are some things you can control and some you can't. You can't fix war, famine, or taxes. They exist. You can feed yourself and make your own decisions (including paying your taxes). Things in green and red are obvious to most people.

What isn't are some of the things that can really bother people in residency (the blue on the edge of the box). The cafeteria isn't open late enough. They don't serve food you can (or want to) eat. The program has decided your clinic and hospital services should be 10 miles apart. That nurse on 2 East won't get the ECG even though you ordered it and told them to do it specifically. The difference between these issues and war or famine is that if you invest enough time and energy into them you might be able to sway influence. But, they require A LOT of time and energy. Further, at the end of an 80 hour week you probably don't have the energy to engage it.

The key to achieving acceptance (Death and Dying In Residency) is to realize what you can and can't change. If you can't change it, tell someone who can; relay it to a superior and move on. Don't fight fights you can't win. But if something needs to be changed and **is in your box, your sphere of influence**, do it.

Also realize that the **higher you achieve in your career the more opportunities come into your box**. As you grow as a person, doctor, and professional you'll slowly begin to expand your sphere of influence. Always be mindful and try to grow your influence, but don't over-extend. Your soul, spirit, and emotional battery just can't handle it. Today you're an intern; it feels awesome (at least I hope it does) to finally be caring for patients. But, right now you can change very little. Don't let it weigh on you.

Remember, in this world the only thing you **can control is YOURSELF**. So, in any situation you find yourself in, the one thing you can to do resolve it is change your attitude.

DOING QUESTIONS

Doing Questions

Questions are for one purpose - beating the test. The Board Exam and USMLE Step 3 **ARE** finite games. Train for the tests, beat them, and move on with your life. They don't matter. They don't test your ability as a doctor, your worth as a person, and certainly not your effectiveness (beyond your ability to take a multiple choice question and regurgitate useless facts).

Here are the rules to the game.
The test writers start with an **educational objective**. That's the clinical question being asked. "Diagnosing Multiple Myeloma," or, "treatment for a CHF exacerbation."

Then they pick a **right answer**. They affix the **appropriate question** to that right answer. Usually this is done in the way of, "what is the best next step in management?"

Then they write **wrong answers**, called **distractors**. A good distractor is one that COULD be right given the right situation. That is to say, if the writer adjusted the vignette in some small way, the wrong answer could become right. It can also be something that sounds attractive to someone who hasn't really studied something, but rather is using loose word association.

From there, they write the vignette. Within it, the vignette contains the diagnosis. **You must first make the diagnosis before you can answer the question**. The question is called the **hinge**. You answer the clinical vignette by determining either the diagnosis or by figuring out where in the diagnostic pathway you are, then you answer the question loosely related to whatever you've diagnosed.

Due to time and space restrictions board exam questions can't be infinitely long. Generally speaking, that means if they **tell you something is there** it's probably useful in making the diagnosis. But here's what's great: if they **tell you something is absent** then that is **most certainly crucial** to the vignette. After all, they don't have space to say all the negatives – if they take the time to say it you can bet it's relevant.

So when doing questions it's not just about, "getting the answer right," or, "reading the explanations." Training for the test is about figuring out how the test writers think. You should at least think about how you would rewrite the vignette to make each of the other answers right. In doing so, you engage the content in greater detail and consider more possibilities from that one vignette.

No. No one who writes for the ABIM also writes review questions.
No. You won't see a question word for word on the ABIM and in a review material.

Yes. Training for test day will let you perform well when you get there; you'll pass the test. When it comes to Finite and Infinite games the Boards are the only finite game you're allowed to play. It'll be your last.

CHAPTER 2: SURVIVAL TECHNIQUES

Studying Resources

1. **Review Book:** This is what you carry with you. It's meant to be glanced at; it's for recall and recognition. Read it at the beginning to highlight what's important. Or, read it at the end to review what you still have to learn. These are First Aid, Step Up, etc. There really isn't anything like this for internal medicine, unless you print out all the "Key Essentials" from MKSAP or Pocket Medicine.
2. **Reading Book:** This is to be fully consumed. It's short enough that you can actually get through it but longer than the review book. It's usually written in complete sentences. It'll begin to round off the edges, but won't bury you. If preparing for boards, use MKSAP17 or MedStudy. If reading for life, I personally recommend Practice and Principles of Hospital Medicine.
3. **Reference Book:** This is the one you'll rarely look at; it sits on your shelf. Its utility is for when you have to do an oral presentation or really want to know EVERYTHING about a topic. Harrison's is a reference book. You won't finish it. If you do, you won't remember it. Should you manage to, you'll know so many inane useless details that you won't be of any use to anyone. You'll hear grey-beards telling you that they, "read Harrison's twice in residency," or, "finished Current's by the end of intern year." They're either lying or it was 1963 when Harrison's was 50 pages and the only antibiotic we had was penicillin.
4. **Journals:** Don't read journals. Two things 1) If I encounter someone who actually knows what they're talking about, I usually just end up saying, "oh, ok," because it's "controversial." Stop reading controversial things. You need to learn foundations, frameworks, etc - leave the journals for after residency is over. True academics will DESPISE this advice. But, what would you rather be - well-read or effective? 2) It's a skill you're likely not ready for. If you must, there are excellent blogs written by people smarter than us that summarize important findings and cover the strengths and weaknesses. Use them.
5. **Questions:** When it comes to learning medical knowledge for life-long success, questions do a terrible job. Some people have conditioned themselves to learn this way and that's ok. If this is you, great. Do questions. That said, when it comes to scoring highly on the Step3 or ABIM exam there's no substitute for questions. A boxer who swims all year may have the cardiovascular endurance to go 12 rounds, but will lack the punching power and fighting ability to win. Thus, you must read for life and do questions for the test. See Doing Questions for more.

Resources

Review	Pocket Medicine		
Reading	MKSAP16	MedStudy	Practice and Principles
Reference	Harrisons	Cecil's	Current's
Questions	MKSAP16		

Board Prep: MedStudy has better READING, MKSAP16 has better QUESTIONS
Life Prep: Practice and Principles of Hospital Medicine

Rounding

and

Documentation

Save yourself some time,
do it right from the start.

Help all those around you
and help them save a life.

"If you don't have time to do it right, when will you have time to do
it over?"
— *John Wooden*

CHAPTER 3: ROUNDING AND DOCUMENTATION

H&P: Spoken Presentation

First Line: State the name, age, gender, and the chief complaint.
- LEAVE OUT past medical history
- Do include radicals and game changers (HIV, Transplant)

First Paragraph: FAR COLDER
- Frequency, Associated Symptoms, Radiation, Character, Onset, Location, Duration, Exacerbating Factors, Relieving Factors
- Tell the attending the timing and characterization exactly as you have it. Give it unadulterated. Let the attending take a second crack at the complaint.

Second Paragraph: This is, by far, the hardest concept to master. Say only what's relevant.

Third Paragraph: What the ED did and what response it had. You may not need this, but if it helps with the differential diagnosis or the understanding of the treatment course, say it.

Review of systems: DO NOT say the words, "review of systems." DO NOT list anything in the review of systems. Anything you thought relevant from the review of systems goes in the second paragraph.

The other stuff:
- PMHx, PSHx, Meds, Allergies, Social, Family
- Get through this as fast as possible; we can look it up later. Refer to it when if asked
- SOMETIMES stuff in here is relevant (debility now, functional status, or you think colon cancer and they had a colonoscopy), but most of the time it's useless. Don't say it.

Physical Exam
- Vitals: Say the numbers. Not, "stable," or, "within normal limits."
  - If they changed, say what they were on presentation followed by what they were when you saw them.
  - If no change, just say what they were at the time you saw them. Again, no ranges during the H&P.
- Physical:
  - Go top down, BUT
    - Say only the things that alter the differential.
    - POSITIVE if there and should be.
    - NEGATIVE if not there and should be.
  - LEAVE OUT the diatribe of normal findings.
  - DO a thorough exam.
  - DOCUMENT said thorough exam.
  - SAY a relevant exam.

H&P: Spoken Presentation

Labs / Imaging:
- Identify abnormals. Don't state normals UNLESS them being negative helps change the differential ("troponin is negative, ECG is normal").
- Lump normals together and summarize: "LFTs and Coags are normal."

Overnight Updates: If you don't talk about a patient the night of admission, but rather are saving it for post-call rounds, this is where you tell us what happened. "That was the original presentation. We thought it was X so we did Y and here is how they've changed."

Assessment:
- DO NOT give a summary. If you have to do so you've failed the presentation.
- DO NOT list their past medical history and chronic conditions in the assessment.
- If the diagnosis is established, clear, and obvious just say what it is.
- If the diagnosis is NOT established and you're still working it up say what is most likely and why. Then list the other diseases it could be and why it isn't.

Plan:
- What you're going to do for the chief complaint.
- List problems and what you're doing in order of acuity and severity.

___

MORE THAN ONE COMPLAINT?
- DO paragraph 1 and 2 for complaint 1
- DO paragraph 1 and 2 for complaint 2 immediately after
- Then go normally
- A/P for problem 1
- A/P for problem 2

NOT A MYSTERY DIAGNOSIS?
If the person comes in with a known complaint, "my doctor told me my hemoglobin was 4," or, "this is my second round of chemotherapy," make these changes:
- First paragraph becomes the history of the disease (not the complaint).
- Skip paragraph two.
- Assessment / Plan becomes what you're going to do and watch for, rather than what the diagnosis might be.

SUMMARY
This is the opportunity to tell everyone about your patient. It's also your opportunity to show everyone how well you understand what's going on. Do this well and you not only look good, but you speed things up on rounds.

A simple case should take **3-5 minutes** (most cases are this).
A standard case should take **5-10 minutes** (the diagnosis is not certain).
A complex case with multiple issues should take **10-15 minutes** (2 a month tops).

CHAPTER 3:   ROUNDING AND DOCUMENTATION

Daily Rounds: Spoken Presentation

BE CONCISE
BE RELEVENT
BE SWIFT (like Taylor)
This should take 30 seconds for simple cases. Two minutes for complex ones.
Use the mnemonic: "iSOAP"

Intro: Who they are and what they're here for: name, age, gender, and diagnosis.

Subjective / Story: The goal is to tell everyone what's happened since the last time the team was together. It's the most variable of all the sections. Your job is to choose what to talk about; it speaks WONDERS of how well you understand your patient's course.
* Interventions started yesterday and the response so far.
* Imaging that led you to make changes in the plan yesterday.
* LEAVE OUT review of systems, incidental complaints, useless information.
* LEAVE OUT imaging and labs that influences your plan for TODAY - that goes in objective.

Objective: This is the data.
* Vital signs: Give a 24-hour range. State them for every patient every time
* Physical exam: Only tell what's relevant for the diagnosis they're here for.
    * Getting better?
    * Getting worse?
* Labs: Don't tell us every lab, just the ones that are relevant for this diagnosis.
* Imaging: Only new imaging not discussed in, "S."
* Culture Data: Every day, whether positive or negative.

Assessment: A one liner
* Very much like the introduction.
    * Name
    * Age
    * Gender
    * THE DIAGNOSIS FOR WHY THEY'RE IN THE HOSPITAL
* Try to utilize CMS language.
* Leave out their chronic medical conditions.

Plan by Problem
* Say what number you're on.
* Give the name of the problem.
* Give the plan for that problem.
* Repeat until plans for all problems are stated.
* ACTIVE ISSUES and SIGNIFICANT DISEASE go first.
What's relevant on the day of admission (the diagnosis) isn't the same thing on day 15 (waiting for placement at rehab). Your presentation must change accordingly.

DOCUMENTATION: SAYING IT RIGHT (FOR CMS)

Documentation: Saying it Right (for CMS)

What you mean to say	What you should write down
There's an infection	Sepsis
Urosepsis	Sepsis secondary to urinary tract infection
Altered Mental Status	Acute Encephalopathy
AKI	Acute Renal Failure
Nausea and Vomiting	Intractable nausea and vomiting
Pain	Intractable pain
Failure of outpatient therapy	Failure of outpatient therapy
The patient's getting better	Resolving
The patient's better	Resolved
The patient's getting worse	Worsening
The patient's probably going to die	Grim prognosis
Any reason that they might need oxygen, in any way, at any time, for any reason. Nasal cannula, CPAP, Intubation, whatever	Acute hypoxemic respiratory failure
Retaining CO2	Acute (or chronic) Hypercapnic respiratory failure
They have a low albumin (<3)	Moderate protein calorie Malnutrition
They have a really low albumin (<2)	Severe protein calorie Malnutrition
The patient is weak	Debility
The patient is weak and from the ICU	Critical Illness Myopathy
CHF exacerbation	Acute or Chronic [HEART FAILURE] with / without exacerbation Systolic/Diastolic Ischemic/Nonischemic Cardiomyopathy with an Ejection Fraction of [EF] New York Heart Association Class
Heart Failure	[1-4]
The troponin elevated and you think it IS an NSTEMI	NSTEMI
The troponin elevated and you think it is NOT an NSTEMI	Demand Ischemia

Whatever you write in the discharge summary overrides and trumps everything you wrote, every day, for the entire stay.

***** If they have something on day one ("sepsis") they must have it on the discharge summary or they never had it at all *****

GET THE DISCHARGE SUMMARY RIGHT WITH THE RIGHT CMS LANGUAGE

CHAPTER 3: ROUNDING AND DOCUMENTATION

H&P: Written Template

Primary Care Physician: First and Last name
Other Physicians: list them and the subspecialty they serve
Chief Complaint: DO NOT quote the patient, say what you are going to address

History of Present Illness:
1. <u>Paragraph 1</u>: FARCOLDER, the timing and characterization of disease.
   a. <u>F</u>requency, <u>A</u>ssociated Symptoms, <u>R</u>adiation, <u>C</u>haracter, <u>O</u>nset, <u>L</u>ocation, <u>D</u>uration, <u>E</u>xacerbating Factors, <u>R</u>elieving Factors
2. <u>Paragraph 2</u>: Review of systems that alter the differential. Try to get two or three questions for each disease on your differential.
3. <u>Paragraph 3</u>: ED interventions and what they found / did. AKA why we're being consulted.

Review of Systems: You can say, *"Thorough review of systems complete and are normal except as listed above."*

Past Medical History: <u>List them</u>, how the diagnosis was made, and when.
Past Surgical History: <u>List them</u>, surgeries with dates. Include scopes caths, etc.
Medications: <u>List them</u> with doses, route, and frequency.
Allergies: <u>List them</u> with reactions.
Family History: <u>List them</u>. Specify mom and dad, other relatives if appropriate.
Social History: <u>List them</u>. Smoking, alcohol, drugs, occupation, living situation, ADLs.

Physical
1. <u>Vitals First:</u> Temperature, blood pressure, heart rate, respiratory rate, oxygen saturation, height, weight, and BMI.
2. Categories: General condition, HEENT, neck, cardiac, pulmonary, gastrointestinal, musculoskeletal, neuro, psychiatry.
3. Goal: at least 3 things per category.

Diagnostics Test: List them and give as much detail as you can.
Laboratory Test: List them and give your INTERPRETATION of the image, do not just copy the report. If you can't do the interpretation yourself, give the gist of the report.

Assessment: A paragraph that lists the chief complaint, your leading diagnosis, and why. Give the information that supports or rejects your differential. Include other diagnoses considered and if they need to be investigated or treated. This SHOULD include a summary of the story, physical, and labs (compared to the oral presentation).

Plan: List out every problem one at a time. For everything that ISN'T the chief complaint, be brief; just list the medications, labs, or whom you're going to talk to. No need to write it all out. That goes into the assessment above.
National Quality Indicators: (see Discharge Summary Template)

54

D/C Summary: Written Template

Primary Care Physician: First and last name

Discharge Diagnoses: <u>List them out</u>. The one you found or fixed should go first. The rest of their history comes next. This is what the next admitting person will use as the, "past medical history," so make it good. You must use ICD code words and speak in the lingo of CMS. <u>Whatever you write here completely overwrites everything you documented in all of your progress notes.</u> You must carry diagnoses from day 1 to the discharge! Even if they get resolved -- if they aren't in your d/c summary, they never happened.

Discharge Medications: <u>List them out</u>. Just give them the list of what you sent them on.

Procedures and Major Tests: <u>List them</u> out.
- Include the date, operator, and procedure name.
- Include major diagnostics (CT, MRI, Echo)
- DO NOT include daily blood tests - these will be in the hospital course by problem.

HPI: Briefly summarize what brought the person in to begin with. Just cover the whole H&P in three or four lines. Finish with, *"please see the H&P for more details."* Every time.

Hospital Course by Problem
- Start with the thing that brought the person into the hospital. The goal here is to provide enough information to let the receiving physician know what happened, but to be short enough so they can actually read it. Don't write a novel, but assure nothing critical is left out. This is where you include lab tests, what you did, and why.
- Go through everything in their discharge diagnosis list. The things you changed or fixed go first. Tell them what you did and why you did it.

Disposition This should be a paragraph. You could list it if you wanted.
- State the <u>condition</u> (good, fair, poor, grim) at discharge.
- State their <u>destination</u>, where they are going (home, rehab, SNF, hospice).
- State any <u>services</u>, what type of care they'll receive (home health, rehab, IV abx).
- State if they if they're a <u>bounce back risk</u>, a <u>death</u> risk, or are to be <u>palliative care</u>.

Followup: <u>List them</u>. Include the Doctor's name, date, and time of appointment.

National Quality Indicators: <u>List them</u>.
- Smoking cessation: Counseling or "Not a smoker"
- Vaccinations: Influenza and Pneumovax
- Code Status: Full, DNR, DNI, modified
- Surrogate Decision Maker: Name, relationship and number
- Core diagnoses: CHF, MI, VTE/PE, CVA, Pneumonia

Time Spent on Discharge: say greater than 35 minutes. It includes Morning Report / Interdisciplinary Rounds, Attending Rounds, Discharge orders, and actually dictating the information.

CHAPTER 3: ROUNDING AND DOCUMENTATION

Ideal Admit Order Set

Admit to: Location, Attending
Diagnosis: What you think your working diagnosis is
Condition: Stable (Obs) / Fair (Floor) / Guarded (ICU) / Guarded (going to die)

Vitals:
 - q1h (unit)
 - q4h (floor)
 - qshift (SNF)
 - qday (NH)
Allergies: List, with reactions.
Nursing: The most open to interpretation. Think about what you want the nurses to do and say it. It might be their routine, but assure more is put down rather than less. Learn from nursing feedback. Different floors have different protocols.
Diet: Diet is chosen based on the problem list as much as the principal diagnosis.
 - NPO
 - Cardiac
 - Renal
 - Diabetic
 - Fluid Restriction.
Activity:
 - Do whatever the patient wants (Ad Lib)
 - Ask PT/OT because you aren't sure (Advance as Tolerated)
 - Stay in the bed (Bed Rest)
 - Fall Precautions
 - Seizure Precautions
Labs: Say what you get and when it's needed by. Be clear; specify a time. You might end up with an LDH (Lactate Dehydrogenase) when what you wanted was a Lactic Acid.
Imaging: Either write what you want or say "none".
Special: Any considerations needed by nursing, or anything that seems out of the ordinary (consent for blood, bring me culture bottles with the paracentesis kit)
Medications: One med per line. Be specific on whether the first dose should be now or later (default is to start tomorrow at 9am). [Name] [Dose] [Route] [frequency].

Consult: PT / OT / ST eval and treat. Write out each consult per line. It's also where to ask for consultants. Pick a specialty or a person.
Call MD if: This tells the nursing staff what they should call you for. They'll call for other things, but if these parameters are met, they WILL call you ~100%.
Contact: your name, number, and hours you work. Also, the name and number (pager is ok) for the people who will be answering questions when you're gone, plus the hours you're out.
Code: Full code, DNR/DNI, or Modified. If modified SPELL IT OUT specifically.

56

Ideal Admit Order Set

As you begin admitting patients with EMR, this may be moot. That's ok. But I want you to see what you're doing and why. Usually, doctors think, "Sepsis, give fluids and antibiotics." The person who actually executes it is the nurse. They need to know what the hell you want and how you want it. Nurses don't make stuff up; they carry out your orders. Make it clear so they can do their job. If it's ambiguous you can expect to receive a multitude of calls.

Admit to: Dustyn Williams, Floor 5B, Telemetry
Diagnosis: Congestive Heart Failure Exacerbation
Condition: Fair

Vitals: q4h
Allergies: NKDA
Nursing: Strict Is and Os, otherwise routine
Diet: <2g NaCl, <2L H20 per day, Cardiac
Activity: ad Lib
Labs:
> AM Labs tomorrow: BMP, CBC no diff
> Stat labs: Troponin, BNP
> Troponin at 2000 (8pm), Troponin at 0400 (4am)

Imaging:
> 2D echocardiogram, indication: CHF

Special:
> Ok to place foley, patient may use urinal

Medications:
> Lasix 80mg IV bid first dose now
> ASA 81mg po qday
> Carvedilol 6.25 mg po bid first dose now
> Lisinopril 40mg po qday first dose now
> Atorvastatin 80mg po qday first dose now

Consult:
> PT eval and treat, prevent deconditioning
> OT eval and treat, prevent deconditioning

Contact:
> Dustyn Williams 987-654-3210 7am-7pm,
> Medicine Group Pager 987-654-0123 7pm-7am

Call if:
> SYS BP > 180 or < 90
> DIA BP > 110
> HR > 120 or < 50
> Temp > 38 or < 36

Code: Do not resuscitate, do not intubate

P.S. That isnt my real cell phone number

CHAPTER 3: ROUNDING AND DOCUMENTATION

Procedure Notes

Sample Procedure Note

Procedure Name:
Procedure Date:
Procedure Indication:

Procedure in detail: take it step by step. Everything you do needs to go in here. See the examples that follow for an idea. Conclude with, "the patient tolerated the procedure well," if there were no complications, or "there was this complication," if there was one.

Appearance of Fluid, if any
Labs / Studies sent on fluid, if any
Blood loss: estimate it. For most medicine procedures it's <5cc.
Lidocaine Used: tell us, in ccs, how much you gave

Operator: (your name)
Supervisor: (if appropriate, generally this is your upper level resident)

Sample Thoracentesis

Procedure name: Diagnostic Thoracentesis
Procedure Date: 5/1/2015
Procedure Indication: Shortness of breath, Pleural effusion

Procedure in detail: Consent obtained from patient after discussing risks and benefits. An ultrasound was used to identify a large pocket of pleural fluid. A mark on the skin was made with a skin pencil. The area was then sterilized once with chlorhexidine. The operator was then dressed in sterile attire, including sterile gloves. The patient was draped.

Using the 25G needle, a small wheal of lidocaine was created. The 25G needle was exchanged for the 18G needle. The track was then anesthetized, approaching the pleural space over the rib. Pleural fluid was encountered and the lidocaine injected. The 5cc syringe was exchanged for the 60 cc syringe. 60 cc of serous fluid was drawn. The 18G needle was then withdrawn and a sterile gauze held in place. A Band-Aid was then placed over the puncture site. The patient tolerated the procedure very well.

Blood Loss: <5cc
Lidocaine use: 5cc

Operator: Dustyn Williams
Supervisor: Dr. Kat

PROCEDURE NOTES

Sample Paracentesis

Procedure Name: Therapeutic Thoracentesis
Procedure Date: 5/1/2015
Procedure Indication: Ascites

Procedure in detail:
Consent obtained from patient after discussing risks and benefits. A pocket of fluid was identified using the bedside ultrasound. The skin was appropriately marked. The operator was dressed in sterile garb. The area was draped with sterile drape. The area was cleaned with chlorhexidine x 3. The 25 gauge needle was used to create an anesthetic wheal. The 25g needle was exchanged for an 18G.The track was anesthetized. Ascitic fluid was encountered. Lidocaine was expressed into the fluid. The 18G needle was withdrawn.

Using the scalpel supplied in the kit, a small nick was made in the skin. Using the stylet, the plastic catheter was introduced into the ascitic fluid. The catheter was advanced into the fluid and the guiding needle withdrawn. Using a one-way valve, the catheter was connected to an external reservoir. Using the 60cc syringe and the one-way valve, 7 liters of serous fluid was removed.

Fluid was not sent for studies.

The patient tolerated the procedure well.

25g IV Albumin was given following the procedure

Blood Loss: < 5cc
Lidocaine Used: <5cc

Operator: Seeyuen Lee
Supervisor: Dustyn Williams

CHAPTER 3: ROUNDING AND DOCUMENTATION

Transfer of Care / Step Down: Written Template

Date of Admit: The day they came in
Date of Transfer: Today's date
HPI: Brief history of the presentation and hospital course so far. Hit the highlights, give a gist of what the person was brought in for and what's happened so far. This isn't as thorough as the hospital course by problem; it should be big picture focused.
Home Meds: List them out.
Current Meds: List them out

Transfer Diagnoses: List them out. Treat this like a discharge summary - include things that are resolved and say they're resolved. The person receiving this note should be able to read it as their discharge. If you did something, and you don't tell the person receiving, they likely won't know or remember to put it in the discharge summary. That means, according to the universe you never did anything.

Procedures and Major Tests: List them out.
- Surgeries, Debridements, I&Ds
- Intubations, Extubations
- Pressors
- Paracentesis, Lumbar Punctures, Thoracentesis, Central Lines
- CT scans, MRIs, Other major imaging

Relevant Labs and trends:
- Culture data (all cultures, including negatives, when and from where)
- Specific labs for the diagnosis (Hgb in GI bleed, Cr in rhabdo)

Today's Labs, Vitals, Review of Systems, and Physical Exam:
Treat it like a regular daily note (this transfer of care COUNTS as the daily note. DON'T write two notes in the same day). Include Plastic (Foley, Central lines, NG tubes, ET tubes).

Hospital Course by Problem WITH PLAN: This is where it gets a little different from a discharge summary. Again, you want to give a brief, non-novel story of what happened with each problem. The ones you are working on go first. Major diagnoses, if resolved, go next. Say what happened, what you did, and why. Then say what you intend to do as if you were going to continue care. List the problems one at a time. You should write 4-5 lines for regular active issues. 10-12 if it's quite complex. 1-2 if it's just a home condition that isn't active. This should match the problem list.

The last problem should be disposition - what it is the barrier to discharge?

Logic: If you followed closely, you'll see it's giving the person all the information to build their data tracker. But most importantly, you're taking what you know about this patient - all the thinking and considerations you've made - and verbalizing them. The goal is let the person taking over act as if they're you, as if you never left, as if the same doctor is taking care of the patient.

60

Medications

Medications are your tools.
It's why it's called "medicine."

Get a handle on the stuff you will see all the time.

Epocrates, Medscape, Uptodate – use them for the weird things you don't often encounter.

Building instinct is crucial.

Refer here for the common medications for the common disorders.

REMEMBER:

"The young physician starts life with 20 drugs for each disease. And the old physician finishes life with one drug for 20 diseases."
– *Osler*

Let's get you somewhere in between.

CHAPTER 4: MEDICATIONS

Meds: Top 50

Drug	Min	Route	Frequency	Type	Notes
Colace	100mg	PO	bid	Hospital	Constipation
Senna	8.6mg	PO	bid	Hospital	Constipation
Bisacodyl	10mg	Rectal	Daily	Hospital	Constipation
Lactulose	20g	PO	prn	Hospital	Constipation
Benadryl	25mg	PO	prn	Hospital	Itching
Zofran	4mg	IV	prn	Hospital	Nausea
Zofran	8mg	PO	prn	Hospital	Nausea
Morphine	2mg	IV	prn	Hospital	Pain
Dilaudid	1mg	IV	prn	Hospital	Pain
Norco	5mg	PO	prn	Hospital	Pain
Norco	10mg	PO	prn	Hospital	Pain
Labetalol	10mg	IV	prn	Hospital	HTN and HR > 90
Hydralazine	10mg	IV	prn	Hospital	HTN and HR < 90

Vancomycin	1g	IV	q12h	Antibiotic	
Zosyn	3.375g	IV	q8h	Antibiotic	
Cipro	400mg	IV	q12h	Antibiotic	
Cipro	500mg	PO	q12h	Antibiotic	
Ceftriaxone	1g	IV	Daily	Antibiotic	
Metronidazole	500mg	IV	q8h	Antibiotic	
Clindamycin	500mg	IV	q8h	Antibiotic	
Azithromycin	500mh	IV	Daily	Antibiotic	
Moxifloxacin	500mg	IV	Daily	Antibiotic	
Nafcillin	1g	IV	q4h	Antibiotic	

Meds: Top 50

Drug	Min	Route	Frequency	Type	Notes
Metoprolol	25mg	PO	bid	HTN Heart	25, 50, 100, 200
Toprol Xl	25mg	PO	Daily	HTN Heart	25, 50, 100, 200
Carvedilol	3.125mg	PO	bid	HTN Heart	3.125, 6.25, 12.5
Lisinopril	40mg	PO	Daily	HTN Heart	2.5, 5, 10, 20, 40
Valsartan	320mg	PO	Daily	HTN Heart	40, 80, 160, 320
HCTZ	25mg	PO	Daily	HTN Heart	12.5, 25
Aspirin	81mg	PO	Daily	HTN Heart	81, 325
Plavix	75mg	PO	Daily	HTN Heart	-
Rosuvastatin	40mg	PO	qHs	HTN Heart	10, 20, 40
Atorvastatin	80mg	PO	qHs	HTN Heart	10, 20, 40, 80
Lasix	40mg	IV	bid	HTN Heart	-

Drug	Min	Route	Frequency	Type	Notes
Tiotropium	18mcg	Inh	Daily	Lungs	
Duoneb	2.5 / 0.5	Inh	q4h prn	Lungs	
ADVAIR	Disk	Inh	bid	Lungs	
PULMICORT	Disk	Inh	bid	Lungs	
Albuterol	90mcg	Inh	q4h prn	Lungs	
Prednisone	40mg	PO	Daily	Lungs	5mg
Guaifenesin	600mg	PO	bid	Lungs	

Drug	Min	Route	Frequency	Type	Notes
Haldol	2mg	IM	prn	Agitation	
Ativan	2mg	IV	prn	Agitation	
Seroquel	50mg	PO	qHs	Agitation	
Zyprexa	10mg	SL	prn	Agitation	

Drug	Min	Route	Frequency	Type	Notes
Lovenox	40mg	SubQ	Daily	DVT	PPx
Lovenox	30mg	SubQ	Daily	DVT	PPx, renal
Lovenox	1mg/kg	SubQ	bid	DVT	Therapeutic
Heparin	5000 U	SubQ	q8h	DVT	PPx
Coumadin	5mg	PO	Daily	DVT	Treatment

CHAPTER 4: MEDICATIONS

Common Meds: Heart Related

Heart Failure

Medications		
Metoprolol Succinate	Start 12.5mg, Max 200mg	Once a day
Metoprolol Tartrate	Start 25mg , Max 100mg	Twice a day
Carvedilol	Start 3.125mg, Max 25	Twice a day
Lisinopril	Start 5, Max 40	Once a day, ACE = ARB
Valsartan	Start 40, Max 320	Once a day, ACE = ARB
Furosemide / Lasix	Start 20, Max 80 (sort of)	Twice a day
Spironolactone	25mg	Once a day
BiDil (Hydralazine / ISDN)	37.5-25 mg	Three times a day

Here you want to max the beta-blocker and the ace-inhibitor before adding on Spironolactone or BiDil. Both Spironolactone and BiDil have one dose. Do not titrate these up in heart failure.

Coronary Artery Disease

Medications		
Metoprolol Succinate	Start 12.5mg, Max 200mg	Once a day
Metoprolol Tartrate	Start 25mg , Max 100mg	Twice a day
Carvedilol	Start 3.125mg, Max 25	Twice a day
Lisinopril	Start 5, Max 40	Once a day, ACE = ARB
Valsartan	Start 40, Max 320	Once a day, ACE = ARB
Aspirin	81 or 325	Once a day
Rosuvastatin	Low 10, Goal 40	Once a day
Atorvastatin	Low 20, Goal 80	Once a day
Clopidogrel (Plavix)	75mg	Once a day

Everyone with coronary artery disease needs to be on Aspirin, Statin, Beta-Blocker, and Ace-i. Other medications are used for anti-anginal properties or blood pressure control. Notice the similarities in the medications for heart failure and CAD.

Hypertension

Medications		
HCTZ	25mg	First Line, Causes Hypo K
Lisinopril	40mg	Causes HyperK, Angioedema, Cough
Valsartan	320mg	Causes Hyper K
Amlodipine	10mg	Anti-anginal, Most expensive cheap HTN med
Labetalol	200mg tid	Only BB for HTN. Use in ESRD
Spironolactone	25mg	Last-ditch, HyperK
Clonidine	0.1 to 0.3 tid	Get your patients off this, it's awful (but works)
Labetalol	10mg IV	If SYSBP >180 AND HR > 90
Hydralazine	10mg IV	If SYSBP > 180 AND HR < 90

Hospital Goal: <180/<110.   **Clinic Goal** varies, but generally <140 / < 80.

COMMON MEDS: LUNG RELATED

Common Meds: Lung Related

COPD

	Medications	
Albuterol	90mcg	
Tiotropium (Spiriva)	18mcg	Once a day
Budesonide/Formoterol	It's a disk, puff twice a day	PULMICORT Bid
Fluticasone/Salmeterol	It's a disk, puff twice a day	ADVAIR Bid
Prednisone	40mg	PO
Albuterol/Ipratropium	2.5 / 0.5mg	q4h prn sob DUONEB
Methylprednisolone	125mg IV	SOLUMEDROL
Doxycycline	100mg PO bid	DOXY

Recognize that the same medications used for outpatient are also used for inpatient exacerbations. You just add on more when an exacerbation happens. To get inpatient criteria, use solu-medrol on admit. Then, rapidly adjust to prednisone after they meet inpatient criteria.

DPE-4 inhibitors exist. Don't memorize them on your common med list.

Asthma

	Medications	
Albuterol	90mcg	
Budesonide/Formoterol	It's a disk, puff twice a day	PULMICORT Bid
Fluticasone/Salmeterol	It's a disk, puff twice a day	ADVAIR Bid
Prednisone	40mg	PO
Albuterol / Ipratropium	2.5 / 0.5mg	q4h prn sob DUONEB
Methylprednisolone	125mg IV	SOLUMEDROL
Magnesium	2g IV	Salvage
SubQ epinephrine	0.1mg SubQ	Salvage

Notice the similarities; the medications are essentially the same. Leukotriene antagonists work basically like inhaled corticosteroids. I don't memorize LTA because it's easier for me to remember the same meds for Asthma as in COPD.

CHAPTER 4: MEDICATIONS

Common Medications: Pain

IV MEDS	Fentanyl Patch →	PO MEDS
Dilaudid		Tylenol
Morphine		NSAIDs
Fentanyl gtt		Tramadol
		Hydrocodone
		Oxycodone
		MS Contin

Short Acting: Everything ~4 hours-ish

Long Acting: MS Contin (PO)
Fentanyl (Patch)

From IV to PCA:

1. Take the total administered IV morphine for a 24 hour period. This is the **total daily dose**.
2. Divide the total daily dose by 24 hours. This is the **basal hourly rate**.
3. Ballpark the **bolus dose:**
   1. If 2mg q4, start with 0.5
   2. If 4mg q4, start with 1
   3. If 8mg q4, start with 2
4. Set the **lockout time:** generally 15 minutes (i.e. there can be 4 pushes every hour)
5. Maintain nursing breakthrough bolus at previous morphine rate

Dilaudid Morphine = MS Contin Fentanyl Oxycodone	Whoa
Hydrocodone Tylenol with Codeine = #3, #4	Scheduled
Tramadol = Mini-opiate Toradol (Super NSAID)	Prescription
Tylenol Advil / NSAID	OTC

- Use an online calculator to convert from one opiate to another
- Morphine 4 = Dilaudid 1
- Oxys are for partying and are abused. Thus, highest schedule
- Hydrocodones are not abused, so are easier to prescribe
- Lortab, Norco = Hydros/APAP
  Percocet, Lorcet = Oxys/APAP
- You can get Oxycodone without Tylenol
  Hydrocodone without Tylenol

66

Common Meds: Poop and Vomit

Constipation

Medications

Colace / Docusate	100mg bid	Stool Softener, Opiate PPx
Senna	8.6mg bid, 17.2mg bid	Motility, Opiate PPx
Lactulose	20mg/30mL prn	Motility, Acute Constipation
GoLytely ®	1 gallon	They will poop

Strength increases as you go down the list. Colace + Senna for opiate induced constipation prophylaxis. Whenever you give a motility agent also give a stool softener. Having lots of contractility against a boulder just hurts.

Other strategies

Your Finger (disimpaction)	Best way to scoop the poop and stimulate the bowel. Do this first before you ask a nurse to do something (below).
Fleet, Soap Suds, Tap Water Enemas	Nurse driven, loosen up some stool. Do after a rectal exam and an attempt at disimpaction.
Lactulose Retention Enema	Put lactulose through a rectal tube (or Foley catheter into rectum). Clamp tube. Let it sit, marinate, and then open it up.

You should disimpact. And by you, I mean the intern. It's a right of passage. Sure it's gross, but it can also save 3-4 days of hospital time just by spending 10 minutes scooping some poop. Do it. Not the ED. Not the nurse. **YOU**.

Emesis

Medications

Diphenhydramine	25mg	When you really don't think they have nausea, but want to give them something.
Promethazine (Phenergan)	12.5 IV, 25mg PO	Start here.
Metoclopramide (Reglan)	10mg IV	Use only in Gastroparesis. Definitely avoid in gastric outlet obstructions. Causes tardive dyskinesia.
Ondansetron (Zofran)	4mg IV, 8mg PO	Strongest we have, technically only supposed to be used for chemo-related nausea.
Dexamethasone	8mg, 10mg, 12mg IV or PO	When nothing else will work.
Lorazepam (Ativan)	0.5, 1mg IV or PO	Adjunct. Don't get in the habit of doing this often.

Strength increases as you go down the list (except lorazepam, which is an adjunct only).

CHAPTER 4: MEDICATIONS

Common Medications: Psych Meds

Sleep & Insomnia

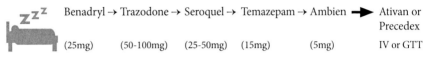

Benadryl → Trazodone → Seroquel → Temazepam → Ambien ➡ Ativan or Precedex

(25mg)   (50-100mg)   (25-50mg)   (15mg)   (5mg)   IV or GTT

EtOH Withdrawal

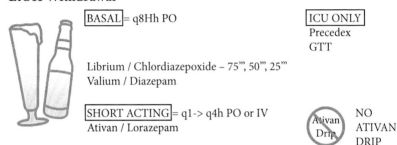

BASAL = q8Hh PO

ICU ONLY
Precedex GTT

Librium / Chlordiazepoxide – 75''', 50''', 25'''
Valium / Diazepam

SHORT ACTING = q1 -> q4h PO or IV
Ativan / Lorazepam

NO ATIVAN DRIP

Standard for prophylaxis: Librium 75mg tid, then 50 tid, then 25 tid with Ativan prn. If they need a lot of prn Ativan, don't decrease the Librium.

For CIWA > 12 (bad withdrawals) put them in the unit with q2H pushes. No drips. There's no maximum Ativan; keep giving it until they're calm.

Anxiety (Acute)

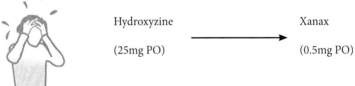

Hydroxyzine ⟶ Xanax

(25mg PO)   (0.5mg PO)

Opiate Withdrawal

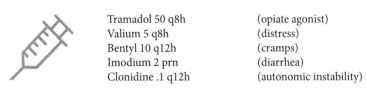

Tramadol 50 q8h   (opiate agonist)
Valium 5 q8h   (distress)
Bentyl 10 q12h   (cramps)
Imodium 2 prn   (diarrhea)
Clonidine .1 q12h   (autonomic instability)

ANTIBIOTICS

Antibiotics

Diagnosis	Empiric antibiotics	Duration
CAP	Ceftriaxone AND Azithromycin or Moxifloxacin	5 days
HAP	Vancomycin AND Zosyn (Linezolid)　　(Meropenem)	5 days
UTI	Ceftriaxone　　(inpatient) or Cipro　　(ambulatory pyelo) or Nitrofurantoin　(cystitis)	3 days for uncomplicated, 7 days for complicated, 10 days for pyelo, 14 days for abscess
Meningitis	Vanc AND Ceftriaxone AND Steroids +/- Ampicillin (immunocompromised)	7 days
Cellulitis	Vancomycin OR Clindamycin (MRSA) Keflex OR Ancef (Strep)	7 days
Diabetic Foot	Vancomycin AND Zosyn	
Diverticulitis	Cipro AND Metronidazole or Zosyn	5-7 days
Cholangitis	Cipro AND Metronidazole or Zosyn	5-7 days

Medications			
Vancomycin	1g	IV	q12h
Zosyn	3.375g	IV	q6h
Zosyn	4.5g	IV	q8h
Zosyn	2.225g	IV	q8h
Cipro	400mg	IV	q12h
Cipro	500mg	PO	q12h
Ceftriaxone	1g	IV	Daily
Ceftriaxone	2g	IV	Daily
Metronidazole	500mg	IV	q8h
Clindamycin	500mg	IV	q8h
Azithromycin	500mg	IV	Daily
Moxifloxacin	500mg	IV	Daily
Nafcillin	1g	IV	q4h

MEDS

Methods

Methods are how you make the diagnosis.

They are the advanced organizers you produce when you have to work through a problem.

They are the framework on which you build illness scripts – the building blocks for your entire career.

Treatments change. Diseases don't (mostly).

You can always look up how to treat something on UpToDate. But knowing what to put in the search field (i.e. the diagnosis) is what separates a master physician from the novice

REMEMBER:

You do a lot of work. You meet core measures. You fill out the H&P flawlessly. Twice. You get all those orders in the system. The patients are educated, counseled, and even rate you highly on your survey (HCAHPS). Great job.

BUT.....

None of it matters if you admit the PE as CHF.

CHAPTER 5: METHODS

Chest Pain

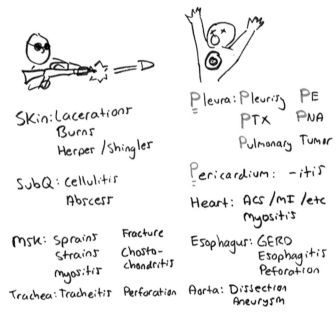

Take a high powered rifle. Aim it at your enemy's chest. Pull the trigger. This is a rifle; it's going through every layer it encounters. In your mind, follow the round as it goes into, through, and out of the chest. What structures does it hit? At each layer, consider what could go wrong with THAT structure.

That's your organizer.

Every patient, every time, has these 10 things asked or done. Every time, regardless of what you think it might be.

1. Where is the pain (going for substernal)?
2. Is it worsened by exertion and relieved by rest?
3. Is it improved by nitroglycerin?
4. Associated symptoms: presyncope, shortness of breath, diaphoresis
5. Risk factors for ACS/CAD: smoking, diabetes, HTN, dyslipidemia, obesity
6. How far can you walk without stopping? What stops you?
7. Is the pain pleuritic?
8. Is the pain tender?
9. Is the pain positional?
10. What's the blood pressure on both arms? Is it the same?

Shortness of Breath

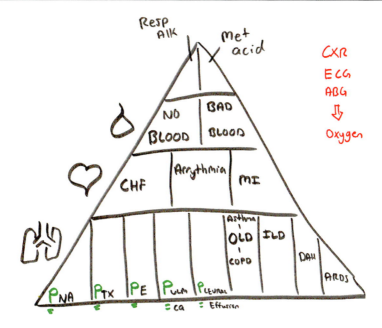

PNA = Pneumonia
PTX = Pneumothorax
PE = Pulmonary embolism
OLD = Obstructive Lung Dz
ILD = Interstitial Lung Dz
DAH = Diffuse Alveolar Hemorrhage

The pulmonary diseases that begin with p can be associated with a pleuritic chest pain because they involve the pleura. The absence of pleuritic chest pain means nothing, however.

"CHF" doesn't distinguish left versus right sided heart failure, ischemic vs non ischemic, tamponade vs effusion or systolic vs diastolic. That's because the signs, symptoms, and tests to order are the same.

When called in the middle of the night, three tests can assess for all diseases except pulmonary embolism. If you don't know what's going on put them on **oxygen** and get:

1. **ABG** – arterial blood gas shows acid base status and hemoglobin
2. **EKG** – assess for ST segment changes + can give information regarding pericardium
3. **CXR** – parenchymal versus extraparenchymal disease

CHAPTER 5: METHODS

Abdominal Pain

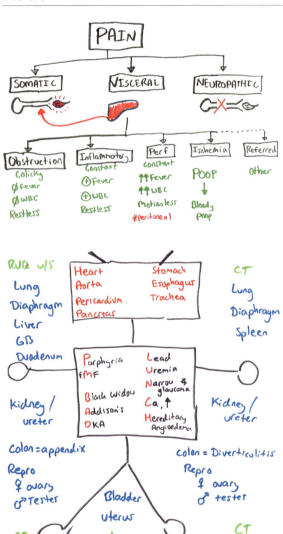

Somatic Pain is pinpoint. The skin or muscle is damaged. It's localizable and often reproducible. The nerve is doing what it's supposed to do.

Visceral pain is vague, diffuse, and occurs as a result of capsular stretch or obstruction of a hollow viscous. Abdominal contents do not feel being stabbed, burned, or cut. Just stretch.

Neuropathic pain is usually described as a burning or pins-and-needles pain. The nerve itself is damaged despite the thing it's innervating being fine. Think of diabetic neuropathy or a radiculopathy.

ABDOMINAL PAIN

Working through the method

The goal's to identify the **type of pain** (somatic, visceral, or neuropathic). If visceral, try to break it down even further using **types of visceral pain**. From there, use the **anatomic location** (the robot) to determine which organs can be involved. Build your differential around those results.

Types of Visceral pain

Obstruction is the blockage of a hollow viscous: bowel, ureter, biliary tree. Peristalsis comes up against the obstruction (which hurts), but then passes it (so it gets better). There's no inflammation , which means no fever or leukocytosis either. The person will be writhing around trying to find a position of comfort. Think nephrolithiasis or cholelithiasis.

Inflammatory will be any organ that's been agitated. There'll be mild fever and leukocytosis. They'll be writhing around trying to find a comfortable position, but they won't find it. Now the pain is constant and won't go away. Think the "–itis" endings: pancreatitis, cholecystitis, pyelonephritis, and diverticulitis.

Perforation is where the patient is **sick as shit**. They'll lie **motionless** for fear that the ruptured contents will shift and touch (painfully) another piece of the abdomen. This manifests as lots of **fever, lots of leukocytosis**.

Ischemic pain presents as **pain out of proportion** (POOP) to the physical exam. Soft belly but intense pain = faking it! Or ischemia.

Referred pain is there to remind us that not all abdominal pain needs a CT. Sometimes the menstruating woman just needs Midol and sometimes that elderly demented guy just needs a rectal. Do a rectal.

Working it up

The **right upper quadrant ultrasound** (one word) is investigated with an **ultrasound**. All other quadrants are going to be investigated by a **CT scan**.

The **epigastric area** and the **chest** are indistinguishable, so consider the organs in the chest (heart attack) for anyone with epigastric pain. Don't work it up everytime, but at least consider it.

Syncope

	Hx + Px		Dx	Tx
Waso Wagal · Visceral Stim · baroreceptors · psychogenic	Recurrent ⊕ Prodrome ⊕ Stimulus	carotid massage Sys BP ↓ 50 Asystole	Tilt Table	Beta Blockers
Orthostatic · Vol ↓ = D/O/O/H · ANS = DM, Age, Parkinsons	orthostatic		IVF	IvF... Steroids?... compression
Mechanical cardiac	Exertional	Murmur	Echo	Surgery
Arrythmia	Sudden ∅ prodrome	NONE	Holter	Cath/CABG
Neurogenic	"	"(FND?)"	Carotid U/S CTA	—
Psych	Faking It	Face-Palm	—	—
E-lytes	—	—	BMP	Replete

Who Gets Admitted?
1. Structural heart disease (CHF, MI, CAD)
2. ECG = Arrhythmia
3. Comorbid reasons (Risk Factors)
   OR
4. Repeat Offenders

Often we observe old people with ortho-statics, "just to make sure," and that's ok. Old people may have coronary artery disease.

Syncope And Seizure

Syncope		Seizure
Short, <30 seconds	Shaking	Prolonged > 30 seconds
Vagal Symptoms	Aura	Smell, Lights, Sounds
< 10 seconds to recovery	Post Ictal	> 30 seconds to recover

What do you order when you admit?
2D Echo
Observation, ECG ("Holter Monitor")
Trend troponins
Carotid Ultrasound is NOT necessary

What about Presyncope?
The run of vtach that caused them to get dizzy this time alerted you to the fact that they may have a slightly longer run of vtach that could cause them to pass out next time.

PRESYNCOPE = SYNCOPE

Weakness

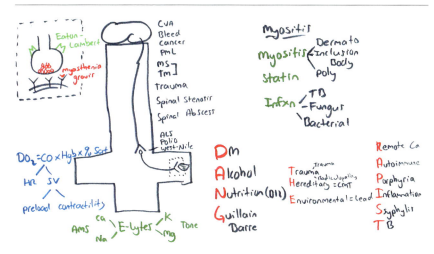

Weakness is broken into multiple categories

1. **Generalized weakness** is the Delivery of Oxygen (**DO**) and the **E-lytes** categories. Delivery of oxygen is from the 10 equations. For electrolytes, Ca and Na generally cause problems with mentation and reflexes, while K and Mg cause problems with tone.

2. **Myositis / Myopathy** are diseases of the muscle itself. If tender, it's myositis. If not, it's myopathy. Think Statin, infection, and autoimmune disease. This can also be steroid-induced or come by way of critical illness myopathy or debility.

3. **Peripheral Neuropathy** is recalled by **DANG THE RAPIST**. Since it involves the peripheral nerve, which carries sensory and motor fibers together, usually both are compromised. For some reason, sensory often predominates in the way of **neuropathy**.

4. **Endplate diseases** like Myasthenia and Eaton-Lambert are in their own class. There are others, but you shouldn't think of them. Just these.

5. **Central Lesions** are a bit tough. Use the anatomic location of the lesion to drive your search. Find where upper and lower motor neuron symptoms predominate. Recall your dermatomes. The brain is usually unilateral, cord is bilateral.

CHAPTER 5: METHODS

Fluid Where Fluid Shouldn't Be (Swelling)

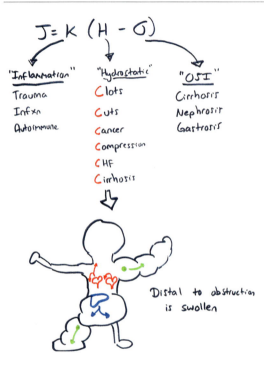

To figure out why there's fluid where fluid shouldn't be, you need to use a bit of physics. The equation, "Jay Equals," has been simplified substantially from your physiology days. This is true in all cases of fluid where it shouldn't be EXCEPT for **pleural effusions and ascites**, where the next step is simply to tap it (not pleural effusions if they have heart failure). So, this simplified version works except when the next step (a tap) is already predetermined.

Inflammation If there's isolated swelling that ignores gravity, it likely involves a **joint** (see approach to joint pain) or a compartment (**hemorrhage**). This is where you should look towards the K part of the equation.

Hydrostatic The Snowman is used to remind you that fluid tends to go **with gravity** and always layers out. That means you can deduce the level of obstruction just by looking at where the swelling is. Start at the left heart and work your way back. If the obstruction is at the level of the left heart, you get fluid in the lungs. If the obstruction is at the level of the right heart, you don't. There would, however, be JVD and both legs would be swollen (since fluid falls with gravity and does so symmetrically).

That also means that if only ONE extremity is swollen and it's asymmetric, the level of the obstruction must be in that one swollen leg. This allows you to hone in on where to look.

OSI Finally, if it's one of the -osi, look for a loss of oncotic pressure (**low albumin**) as a tipoff to send you down the -osi route. This is because the liver can't build the albumin (cirrhosis), the protein is being lost in the urine (nephrotic syndrome, "nephrosis") or because there's a GI problem (gastrosis). GI problems are either Kwashiorkor malnutrition or it's a protein-losing enteropathy such as pernicious anemia.

78

Delirium

"HE STOPS FOR TIPS ON VOWELS"   HE STOPS TIPS AEIOU

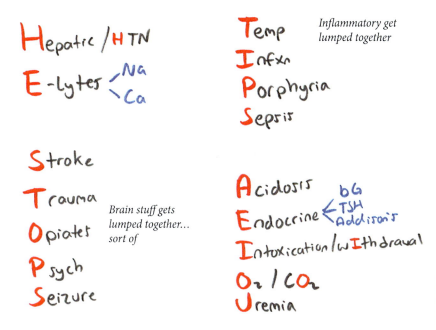

Hepatic / HTN
E-lytes — Na, Ca

Stroke
Trauma
Opiates
Psych
Seizure

Brain stuff gets lumped together… sort of

Temp
Infxn
Porphyria
Sepsis

Inflammatory get lumped together

Acidosis
Endocrine ← bG, TSH, Addisons
Intoxication / wIthdrawal
O_2 / CO_2
Uremia

When patients are altered getting a history can be tough. It's great when there's a bystander or family member to help, but often that's not a luxury we have, or their history is everything up to the time where you actually need the information. After all, the patient generally can't tell anyone what's going on when altered.

So you rely on veterinarian medicine.

A lot goes into the physical exam and the labs. Their medical history, whether known or inferred from their medications, goes a long way.

CHAPTER 5: METHODS

Hemoptysis

Bronchiectasis / Bronchitis

Aspergillus / Autoimmune

TB

Tumor

Lung Abscess

Embolism — Air
  — Placenta
  — DVT / PE
  — Fat / Cholesterol

Cystic Fibrosis / Coagulopath

AVM / DAH

Mitral valve

Pneumonia

Bronchitis and Pnuemonia are the most common.

TB, Tumor, and Trauma (coughing from cancer of infection) are "classically" associated with hemoptysis.

Assure you're able to separate **hematemesis** (call GI) from **hemoptysis** (call pulm). This should be obvious, but it requires actually probing patients to get the information. Don't accept that their words are meaningful. Hear the complaint then ask it specifically: cough or vomit?

If you're in **hemoptysis** also consider where this is. Is it **lung** (call pulm) or **oropharynx** (call ENT)?

80

Fever

House Method

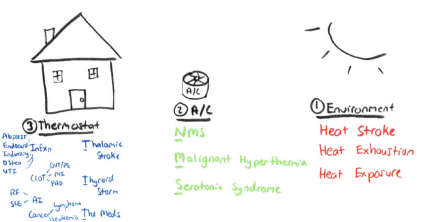

There are three different ways of getting an **elevated temperature**. While this section is fever, the focus is really about **hyperpyrexia** of any kind. Don't miss anything! Use the "House Method" to organize. It's separated into the sun, cooling system, and thermostat.

1. **Environment:** Environmental exposure can cause elevated temperatures, dehydration, and altered mental status. Look for the red flushed look, exposure to extreme heat, or prolonged time without access to water / cool environment.

2. **Cooling System.** Dysregulation of the cooling system can cause an increase in the amount of heat produced. That is, the body doesn't want to be this hot; the heat is coming from within. Think of the mnemonic "NMS".

3. **Increased thermostat.** Inflammation sets the temperature a bit higher than it normally is. **Inflammation** of any kind does so by influencing the hypothalamus via IL-1. Infections are in this category, but so are clots, autoimmune disease, cancer, and some weird stuff: Thalamic Stroke, Thyroid storm, The meds. Just remember,

"FEVER = INFECTION" is for med students. "FEVER= INFLAMMATION" is for you.

CHAPTER 5: METHODS

AKI

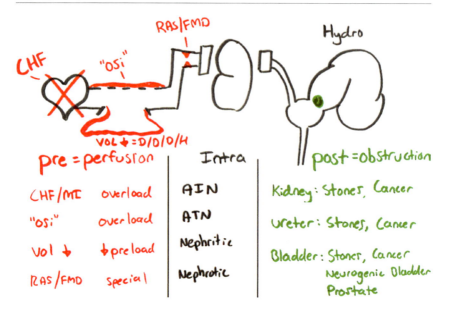

Start by dividing the kidney into three distinct regions. Then, further subdivide into individual diagnoses.

1. **PRE RENAL** means **DECREASED PERFUSION** for any reason. It doesn't matter whether the pump is broken (CHF, MI) or the pipes are broken (Vol Down = Diarrhea, Dehydration, Diuresis, and Hemorrhage), are leaky ("Osi" – nephrosis, gastrosis, cirrhosis, cardosis), or have clogged (Renal Artery stenosis, fibromuscular dysplasia). The response will be the same.

2. **POST RENAL** means **OBSTRUCTION**. Obstruction blocks the flow of urine. The kidneys try to make urine. More into a balloon without any out of the balloon means the balloon swells. This is called **hydro**, either **hydroureter** or **hydronephrosis**. The level of obstruction determines what the urinary system will look like. **Stones and cancer** are always considerations, but so too are things like a **neurogenic bladder** or **BPH** leading to outlet obstruction.

3. **INTRA RENAL** disease is the final division and can be quite confusing. It could be ATN, AIN, Glomerulonephritis, Nephritic, Nephrotic, or progression of chronic kidney disease. Rarely will you go here, so focus instead on PRE and POST renal.

AKI

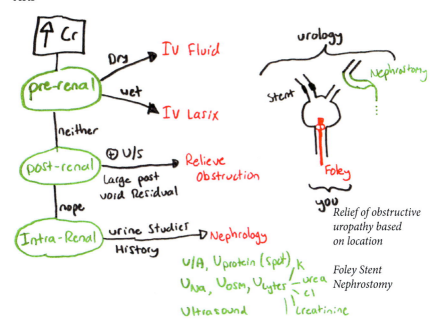

How we actually investigate renal failure is much different than you'd expect.

Start with what's most likely; the majority of the answer will come from the **history and physical**. You DON'T need a FeNa or a BUN/Cr ratio. The story, almost always, provides the answer rather than the lab tests.
1. Are they overloaded, have heart failure, and edema to their nipples? Give lasix
2. Are they septic, borderline shock, and happen to have an elevated creatinine? Give fluids
3. Does the patient have MS, a distended, painful bladder, and the inability to void? Put in a Foley

However, there will be times that you aren't sure what to do. So, start at the top and work your way down. Keep in mind that if you're going to call nephrology, you need to have some answers first:
1. Ultrasound
2. Urine studies: lytes including Na, K, Cl, Creatinine, and Urea
3. Urinalysis
4. Spot Protein (where appropriate)

CHAPTER 5: METHODS

Bleeding

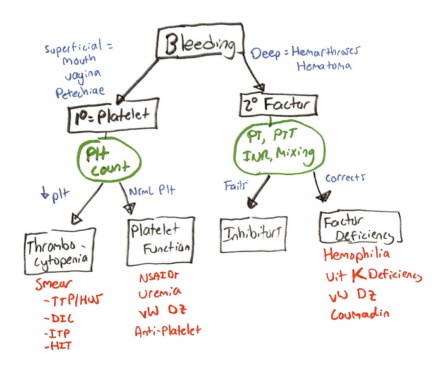

The first step is to separate the bleeding into **primary hemostasis** (problems with **platelets**) and **secondary hemostasis** (problems with **factors**). To do that, see bleeding as either **superficial** (primary hemostasis is broken, presenting with petechiae, gingival bleeding, and vaginal bleeding) or **deep** (secondary hemostasis is broken, presenting with hemarthrosis and hematomas).

Regardless of which branch you're in, the decision is if there's a **deficiency** or an **inactivation**. This happens in different ways in each branch, but it's crucial to determine if 1) there are enough platelets (CBC) and 2) if there are enough factors (mixing study). Once you're into one of the four final buckets it's time to begin thinking of a broader list. This is a good starting place.

It's **OK** to just get both a **CBC AND INR** when someone comes in bleeding more than they should.

84

Dysphagia

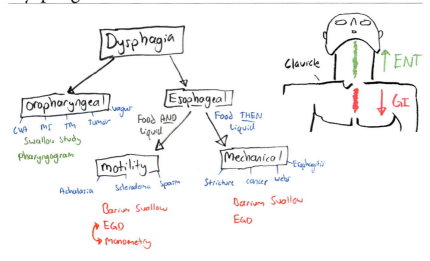

Dysphagia is trouble swallowing. Not pain.
Odynophagia is painful swallowing and has a different (and separate) differential.

Step 1: Oropharyngeal or Esophageal?

If the food gets stuck **above the clavicle (ENT, Speech)** it's probably an oropharyngeal problem. GI can't help you. If the food gets stuck **below the clavicle (GI)** it's likely to be an esophageal problem. Yay, GI can help you.
But oropharyngeal dysphagia can present with more than food getting stuck. If there's coughing, choking, or literally ANYTHING on **initiation of swallow** then it's an oropharyngeal problem. Most problems with the oropharynx are neuromuscular in nature; you should give consideration to demyelinating diseases and stroke. **Speech therapy** and their **pharyngogram** is where you want to go to work this up.

Step 2: It's Esophageal, now is it motility or mechanical?

Mechanical is better named **obstructive**. Something grows into the lumen and gets in the way. Since it grows over time the patient will describe dysphagia first to solids (large caliber) **THEN** liquids (smaller and smaller caliber until liquid is a problem).

Motility is better named **functional**. Peristalsis is lost as the esophagus doesn't behave the way it's supposed to. Because it has nothing to do with an obstruction, the caliber of the food doesn't matter. Thus, the patient will describe dysphagia to liquids **AND** solids.

Both Esophageal forms are diagnosed first with a **barium swallow** followed by **EGD**.

CHAPTER 5: METHODS

Back Pain

Admit and Imaging

Most back pain is **musculoskeletal** (like 90%) and doesn't need advanced imaging or intervention. It'll respond to symptomatic anti-inflammatories and stretching (NSAIDS + Mild Exercise) within **2-4 weeks**.

Identifying which patients need admission and immediate imaging becomes crucial. Anyone with **red flags** warrants imaging. Anyone with a **new focal neurologic deficit** gets both **steroids + imaging**. They'll also likely need to intervened upon, and soon.

- Admit red flags
- Image red flags
- Steroids and call surgery for people with acute cord compression

Worry about Acute Cord Compression

- Loss of bowel, bladder function
- Inability to walk because of weakness
- Loss of motor or sensation

Imaging

X-rays are usually useless. They show **normal anatomical variants** that may be, "abnormal," but aren't contributing to pain.

CT scans are used to image bone. Use CT when looking for fracture, or if you need a myelogram and MRI isn't available.

MRI is the best way to evaluate the back. What you care about is nerve impingement. Only the MRI can see the cord / nerves.

Visceral	Pancreas Aorta Hematoma Kidneys Uterus	Pain not elicited with movement or palpation
Spine	Fracture Abscess Osteomyelitis Pott's Mets	Percussive tenderness
Nerve	Herniation Osteophytes Spinal Stenosis Cauda Equina Spondylolisthesis	Worsened by stretch (leg-lift)
MSK	Strain Sprain Overuse	Belt-like pain
Auto Immune	Ank Spond RA Other seronegatives	Associated with arthritis

Red flags

*** Focal Neurologic Deficit ***

Fever (infectious)

Percussive Tenderness (fracture)

H/O Cancer (mets)

Coagulopathy (hematoma)

Immunosuppression (infectious)

Spinal Procedure (abscess, hematoma)

Headache

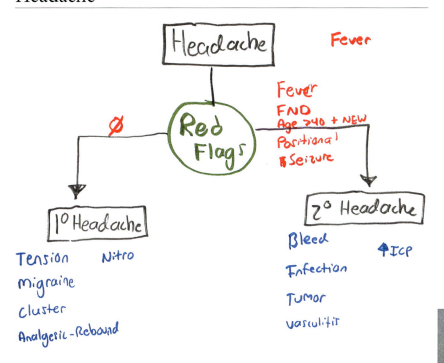

The differential for headache can be quite laborious. The first step is to decide if it's a **primary parenchymal headache** or an extrinsic **secondary headache**. Do that by looking for the **red flags** (listed in red/on yes path above). They're signs that this might be something more sinister.

In general, **secondary headaches** need **imaging and intervention immediately** while primary headaches can be treated medically. Some evidence says that Cluster and Migraine headaches need imaging too, but we're not sure 100%. Even if you diagnose one of these vascular primary headaches, the imaging is a ONE-time thing; not each time they show up to the ED.

"Cluster" actually means trigeminal cephalgias, of which there are three forms: SUNCT, SUNA, and Cluster. Don't memorize them; simply realize there are more than just cluster and they're based on the duration and frequency of attacks. That's beyond an intern level discussion – it's more important that you have the differential at this point.

CHAPTER 5: METHODS

Joint Pain

Determining the diagnosis of joint pain is multi-faceted.

The first consideration is the **number of joints involved**; it's the basis for the organizer. Not that infectious arthropathies or crystal arthropathis CAN'T be monoarticular, it's just that they're likely to present with multiple joints. If it's not multiple joints at THIS presentation, it eventually will be over the course of the patient's disease and show in more than one joint.

The second is **toxicity and acuity**, which parallel each other. The more toxic a disease, the more acute it will be. Toxic and acute diseases cause loss of function, painful swollen joints with deformity, and a high fever. The patient will seek your attention. The less toxic disease (and the more insidious ones) will present with weight loss, night sweats, low grade fevers, and possibly a barely problematic joint. Knowing which diseases present in which way can help you separate them.

The third is **which joint is involved**. This helps the least, but there are some diseases that have a predilection for certain joints. For example, RA attacks little joints like the hands and feet, OA affects the large weight bearing joints, and Ank Spond attacks the spine. You have to know the details of each disease to use this information, which is why it's the least useful of the three.

Diarrhea

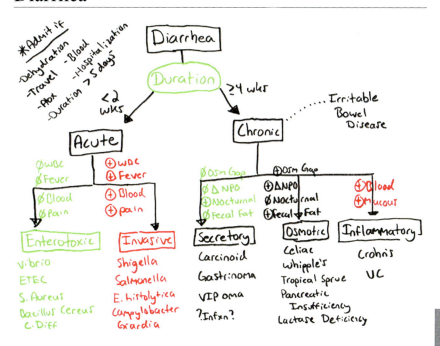

Acute diarrhea (<2 weeks duration) is "always" infectious. The goal is to determine if there's **enterotoxic diarrhea** (no invasion so no leukocytosis, fever, or blood) or if it's **enteroinvasive** (yes invasion so leukocytosis, fever, and blood). The causes of each are broad and listed above.

In the United States, most of the time diarrhea is going to be **viral and self-limiting**. You should look for **nausea, vomiting and diarrhea**. If there's, "vomiting from both ends," it's going to be gastroenteritis.

If not, or if any of the above "Admit If" criteria are met, they'll need an admission, fluids, and a stool workup.

Chronic Diarrhea (>4 weeks) can be, but rarely is, infectious. The key here is to separate it into **secretory, osmotic, and inflammatory** based on the presence of an osmolar gap / fecal fat, nocturnal symptoms, and a response to NPO. If at any time there are blood or white cells in the stool, it's inflammatory.

Irritable bowel syndrome has traditionally been a diagnosis of exclusion.

CHAPTER 5: METHODS

Pulmonary Hypertension

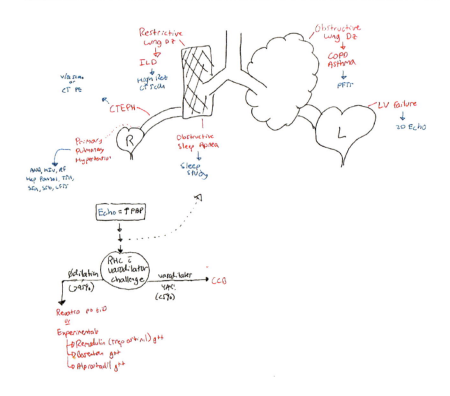

The way cardiologists see pulmonary hypertension is, "oh, the echo shows pulmonary hypertension… some stuff happens… let's do a RHC!"

At that right heart cath the cardiologist will attempt a vasodilator challenge. It works - YAY, you win. Use calcium channel blockers. It doesn't - BOO, you lose. Use Revatio and experimental drugs.

The idea is that the original insult causes the pulmonary pressures to go up. The right heart pumps harder to accommodate. The pulmonary artery gets thicker to accommodate the RV. Intervene before that becomes permanent.

The "some stuff happens" is where you come in.

The organizer is two sides of the heart, separated by two diseased lungs. Start on the right side of the page and work your way left, from the left heart through the lungs to the right heart.

PULMONARY HYPERTENSION

First, let's talk about **the left ventricle**. Heart failure, whether diastolic or systolic leads to increased pressures. Diagnose heart failure with an **Echo**. It's called, "pulmonary venous," in Harrison's.

The lung, "primary parenchymal," in Harrison's, can have a couple of things wrong with it. But it's all hypoxemic lung disease. Hypoxia causes vasoconstriction in the lung. Hypoxemia everywhere means vasoconstriction everywhere, which means higher pressures. Any hypoxemic lung disease can do it, but it must be chronic. **COPD** is diagnosed with **PFTs, interstitial lung disease** is diagnosed with a **high res CT scan**, and **Obstructive Sleep Apnea** is diagnosed with a sleep study.

The last thing to consider is "primary artery." The only disease you can do anything about is **Chronic Thromboembolic Pulmonary Hypertension (CTEPH),** diagnosed with **CT PE** or **V/Q**.

If nothing pops, it's **primary pulmonary hypertension**. Incidence of this is about 1:million.

At this point you must do a thorough investigation of the weird stuff. Get an ANA, HIV, Hepatitis Panel, RF, Anti-Scl70, Anti-centromere, and LFTs. You're questing for some really weird stuff at this point.

CHAPTER 5: METHODS

ECG Interpretation

Three Lead = Rhythm diagnosis?

Look at the rhythm strip. Ignore the 12-lead part; just get the rhythm first.

1.	Regular or Irregular	*line up the R to R intervals*
2.	Rate	*use the 300-150-100-75-60-50-40-30 rule*
3.	PR interval	*does it change, is it long (>.20, one big box)*
4.	QRS complex	*is it wide (>0.12, 3 little boxes) or narrow*
5.	P for every QRS	*just make sure there is one*
6.	QRS for every P	*just make sure there is one*

Major Diagnoses: And Treatment
Fast Ventricular Issues

– Vtach	Amio	Shock	
– Vfib	Amio	Shock	
– Torsades	Amio	Shock	Mag

Fast Atrial

– Afib	CCB = BB	Shock
– Aflutter	CBB = BB	Shock
– SVT	Adenosine	Shock
– S. Tach	fix the underlying problem and please don't shock this (Serial)	

Slower

– S. Brady		
– 1st Degree Block	Atropine	Pace
– 2nd Degree Block, I	Atropine	Pace
– 2nd Degree Block, II	Atropine	Pace
– 3rd Degree Block	No atropine	Pace
– Idioventricular	No atropine	Pace

ECG Interpretation

Vtach:

Vfib:

Torsades:

Afib:

Aflutter:

SVT:

S Tach:

S Brady:

1st Block:

2nd Type 1:

2nd Type 2:

3rd Block:

Idioventricular:

Asystole:

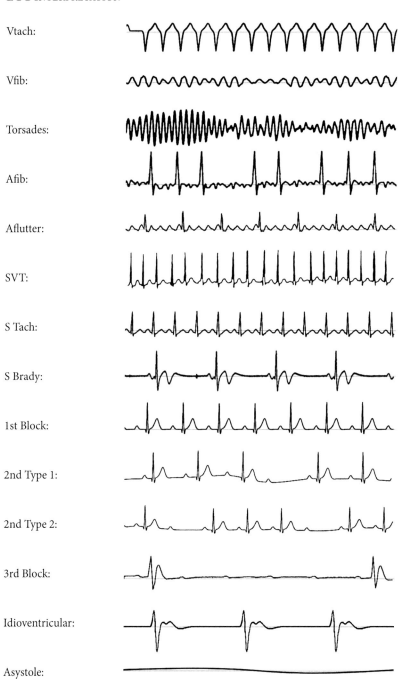

METHODS

chapter 5:   Methods

Twelve Leads

Then Look at the 12 lead:
1. **Axis**
    – Thumb method
        – How to set it up
            – Left thumb = Lead I
            – Right thumb = Lead aVF
        – How to interpret
            – Left up, Right up = Normal Axis
            – Left up, Right down = rocket to the left = LAD
            – Left down, Right up = rocket to the right = RAD
            – Both down = whoa = EXTREME LAD

2. **T-waves**
    – Lead to Location
        – II, III, aVF = Inferior
        – V1, V2 = Septal
        – I, V5, V6 = Lateral
        – V1-V4 = Anterior or Posterior
    – What the T-wave Means
        – Ischemia (flipped T)
        – Infarct (ST elevation)
        – Dying (Q wave with ST elevation)
        – Too Late (Q wave, ST resolved)

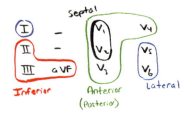

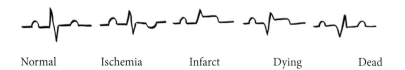

   Normal   Ischemia   Infarct   Dying   Dead

3. **LVH**
    – Add [V1 or V2] to [V5 or V6]... if >35 you got it

4. **Other stuff.**
    – Ok. There's more than this; don't worry about it. You aren't a cardiologist.

Cough

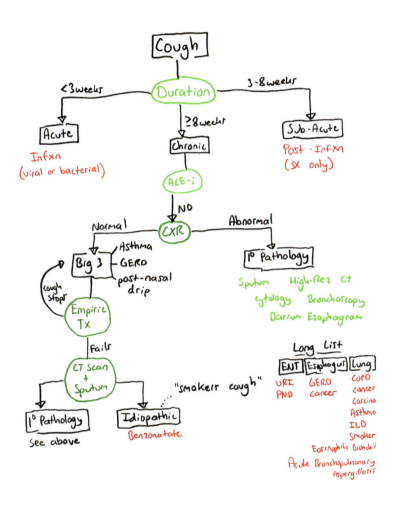

CHAPTER 5:   METHODS

Acid Base and the Chamber of Secrets

When you pull out an ABG you get overwhelmed. Admit it and the rest of this will go easier. Here's how to handle ABGs the right way:

1.   Don't use ranges. Normal **pH 7.4**. Normal **pCO2 40**. Normal **Bicarb 24**, ignore pO2.
2.   Don't use the Bicarb on an ABG, use it on the BMP.
3.   Don't use the word "compensation"; you'll make errors. Changes are either appropriate or not appropriate. If you say the word compensation, I will slap you.
4.   Say "Bicarb" and "CO2" because the Bicarb on a BMP looks like CO2.
5.   Pick a chamber. Run through it. Leave the chamber only when you reach the end, and, only if you're supposed to.

Playing the game

- Step 1:   pH: acid or base
- Step 2:   pCO2: respiratory or metabolic
- Step 3:   Is there another disturbance? This varies by chamber

Primary Disturbance (the one that's winning)

Two things are needed to determine the primary disturbance: the pH and the pCO2, both from the ABG. If you remember that CO2 is a respiratory acid, it can be determined which of the four acid base disturbances is predominating just by looking at the pH and the pCO2 This is Step 1 and 2 of "Playing the Game."

This puts you into a chamber. Once in a chamber, run it through to the bottom.

If the pH is < 7.4, it's an **acidemia**.
   If that acidemia is caused by the respiratory acid, then we'd expect the CO2 to be high. So, if the pH is < 7.4 and the pCO2 > 40, it's **respiratory acidosis** (chamber 1).

   If that acidemia is not caused by the respiratory acid, then we'd expect the CO2 to be low. So, if the pH is <7.4 and the pCO2 < 40, it's **metabolic acidosis** (chamber 2).

If the pH is > 7.4, it's an **alkalemia**.

   If that alkalemia is caused by respiratory acid, that would mean we had too little acid, so the CO2 should be low. If the pH is >7.4 and the CO2 <40, it's **respiratory alkalosis** (chamber 3).

   If that alkalemia is NOT caused by the respiratory acid, then we'd expect the CO2 to be high. So, if the pH is >7.4 and the pCO2 > 40 (it wasn't what we expected for a respiratory alkalosis), by default it's **metabolic alkalosis** (chamber 4).

ACID BASE AND THE CHAMBER OF SECRETS

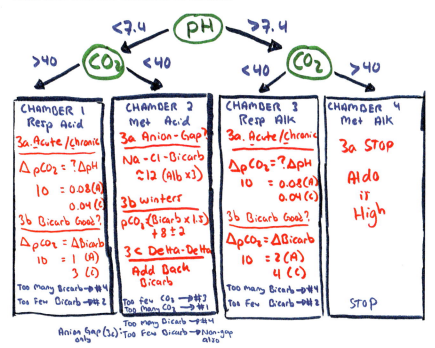

Practice. Run the silos on as many ABGs as you can. The answer **can't** be seen from the beginning; you must go through the whole process every time. Yes, you'll feel silly playing with number like 7.36, but do it anyway. Perfect practice makes perfect.

CHAPTER 5: METHODS

Run The Chambers

Chamber 1: Respiratory Acidosis

> 3a. Acute or Chronic
> 3b. Bicarb appropriate or not

For every "dime change" (**pCO2 of 10**) the **pH** should change by **.08 if acute** and **.04 if chronic**. So, determine what you think the pH should be based on the pCO2 from the ABG. Calculate the change in pH for both acute and chronic. Compare both calculations to your actual pH. Whichever is closest is what it actually is (acute or chronic).

For every "dime change" (**pCO2 of 10**) the **bicarb** should change by **1 if acute** and **3 if chronic**. Normal bicarb is 24. Determine what the value should be for the pCO2 on the ABG. In respiratory acidosis, the pCO2 rises, so the bicarb decreases to compensate (SLAP!). So for every "dime change" subtract 1 if acute, 3 if chronic bicarbs from 24. This is your **expected bicarb**. Compare your expected bicarb to the actual bicarb on your BMP. If there are too few bicarbs (your bicarbs on the BMP are less than expected) it's an additional metabolic acidosis (go to chamber 2). If there are too many bicarbs it's an additional metabolic alkalosis (go to chamber 4).

Chamber 3: Respiratory Alkalosis – *same as Chamber 1, except 2 and 4 instead of 1 and 3.*

> 3a. Acute or Chronic
> 3b. Bicarb appropriate or not

For every "dime change" (**pCO2 of 10**) the **pH** should change by **.08 if acute** and **.04 if chronic**. So, determine what you think the pH should be based on the pCO2 from the ABG. Calculate the change in pH for both acute and chronic. Compare both calculations to your actual pH. Whichever is closest is what it actually is (acute or chronic).

For every "dime change" (**pCO2 of 10**) the **bicarb** should change by **2 if acute** and **4 if chronic**. Normal bicarb is 24. Determine what the value should be for pCO2 from the ABG. In respiratory alkalosis, the pCO2 falls, so the bicarb increases to compensate (SLAP! SLAP!). So for every "dime change" of pCO2, add 1-if-acute, 3-if-chronic bicarbs to 24. This is your **expected bicarb**. Compare your expected bicarb to the actual bicarb on your BMP. If there are too few bicarbs (your bicarbs on the BMP are less than expected) it's an additional metabolic acidosis (go to chamber 2). If there are too many bicarbs it's an additional metabolic alkalosis (go to chamber 4).

ACID BASE AND THE CHAMBER OF SECRETS

Chamber 2: Metabolic Acidosis

      3a. Anion Gap or not
      3b. Winters' Formula (is the Co2 appropriate or not)
      3c. Delta-Delta or Add Back (is there another metabolic disturbance)

The first thing to do is determine if there's an **anion gap**. The normal gap is "12." The easiest way to calculate a normal anion gap is albumin * 3. This is also an estimate. Use Alb * 3 and call it the expected gap.

Na - Cl - Bicarb = Actual Gap. There's an **Anion Gap** if **Actual Gap > Expected Gap**.

Separately, use the Winters' Formula to see if there's an additional respiratory disturbance. If the **actual pCO2** (from the ABG) is within the range of the **calculated pCO2** (winter's) then there isn't an additional disturbance. If there are too many pCO2 (actual > calculated) then it's an additional respiratory acidosis (go to chamber 1). If there are too few pCO2 (actual < calculated) then it's an additional respiratory alkalosis (go to chamber 3).

Lastly (and this step is unique to Anion Gap Met Acid), you have to find out if there's yet another acid base disturbance. To do that, use the **add back method**. There's an anion gap. Find out "how many acids had to be added to get there." (Actual Anion Gap - Expected Anion Gap). Because bicarb and H+ come out of solution in 1:1 ratio, that represents how many bicarbs had to come out of solution to yield this current gap. Add that number to the reported bicarb on the BMP. This is your calculated bicarb.

If calculated bicarb > 24 (normal) there are too many bicarbs. This means an additional metabolic alkalosis (chamber 4).

If calculate bicarb < 24 (normal) there are too few bicarbs. This means an additional non-anion-gap metabolic acidosis.

If calculated bicarb is normal, there's no additional metabolic disturbance.

Chamber 4: Metabolic Alkalosis

      3a. Aldo is high. Stop

Really. Stop. You can do some stuff. By why? Just. Don't. Do. It.

Except make sure there's no anion gap; don't miss an anion gap.

Common Medical Problems

The Medicine.

The Patient Care.

Finally! It's what I've always wanted to do!

Get good at the usual stuff so you can focus on the unusual.

Master this material, Cultivate the rest.

CHAPTER 6:   COMMON MEDICAL PROBLEMS

Cardiac Chest Pain

Is it cardiac chest pain? The only thing you care about in inpatient medicine when someone says "chest pain" is, "is it coronary ischemia or not." After getting past that, you can work on the details: what it is and what has to be done.

Let's go into this: nature of the chest pain, associated symptoms, risk factors, and labs.

Diamond Classification Use the right terminology. The more you have on the Diamond Classification, the more likely you have cardiac chest pain. Atypical doesn't mean unusual. Typical doesn't mean classic. They mean:

Diamond Classification	
3/3	Typical
2/3	Atypical
<2/3	Non-anginal
1.	Substernal Chest Pain
2.	Worsened by Exertion
3.	Relieved by Nitroglycerin

Risk Factors These are ranked by the order in which they increase the risk, top down (most to least, though still important).

Risk Factors
Vasculopathy
Diabetes
Smoking
Age: M > 45, W > 55
Dyslipidemia
Hypertension
Obesity

Associated Symptoms You want to know about poor perfusion to essential organs (like the heart, lung, and brain).

Associated Symptoms
Dyspnea
Diaphoresis
Presyncope

Physical Exam No physical exam finding other than evidence of new heart failure speaks FOR a heart attack. These maneuvers suggest another disease, though an MI can still present with these findings.

Physical Exam
Positional
Pleuritic
Tender

And for CHF or Vascular Disease:

CHF	Vascular Disease
JVD	Aortic Stenosis
Crackles	Carotid Bruit
S4	↓ Distal Pulses
S3	Stigmata of PVD

Labs An elevated **troponin** is indicative of an **NSTEMI** (it's "real" when >1.0)

ECG changes are bad. ST-Elevations or new LBBB are indicative of a **STEMI**

T-wave inversions, ST depressions, and new arrhythmia are suggestive of ischemia, but don't constitute a STEMI.

You can't think so you just plug and chug NOT NSTEMI, NOT STEMI, and NOT something else non-cardiac. TIMI SCORE The timi score tells you the mortality risk IF this is a cardiac chest pain. It does not help you decide "cardiac" or "not cardiac"

Characteristics	Pt	Score	Risk
Age > 65	1	0-1	5%
≥ 3 Risk Factors	1	2	8%
Known CAD	1	3	13%
ASA in 7 days	1	4	20%
ST dev ≥ 0.5 mm	1	5	26%
Cardiac Markers	1	6-7	41%
Severe Angina	1		

102

So you admitted that chest pain

Treatment for coronary ischemia
Ok. It's NOT a STEMI (that goes to the cath lab) but you want to know what to do with them while they are here. Everybody gets MONA BASH.

M	Morphine	B	Beta Blocker
O	Oxygen	A	Ace-Inhibitor
N	Nitro	S	Statin
A	Aspirin	H	Heparin

Here are some decisions to make:

Heparin: how much do we give to this patient? A **therapeutic dose** (1mg/kg Lovenox BiD) is given because you truly believe it's ACS. A **prophylactic dose** (40mg Lovenox) is administered because they're coming into the hospital and everyone needs DVT prophylaxis.

Plavix: do you Plavix load? Plavix is given 75mg daily. A Plavix load is 600mg x 1. Here's the fun game: if you think they can be fixed by cath, give Plavix load. If you think they'll need CABG, then don't, as they'd have to wait 5 days for the Plavix to wear off to go to CABG. How do YOU, the hospitalist, know that it's multi vessel disease or not? Yeah… you don't.

Here's what you do: if you're pretty sure **it's coronary ischemia** (either troponins are elevated <u>OR</u> you're so sure that it's cardiac that you're going to call cards in the morning without a stress test) then give full dose anticoagulation and Plavix load.

If they're coming in for a **rule out** and you think it's garbage, don't do Plavix or full dose heparin, just do MONA BASH.

So you want to rule them out
Admit them to telemetry (people with ACS die from arrhythmias), give MONA BASH, and keep them NPO. Then cycle troponins and ECGs. No Need for CKMB here. No therapeutic lovenox, no plavix load.

ECGs	q6h x 3 (or until ST ↑)
Troponins	q6h x 3 (or until they peak)
Stress Test	See below

They ruled out, now what?
Well, either you knew they didn't have coronary ischemia and you just admitted them because the ED told you (discharge) or they just didn't have an MI in front of you (needs further evaluation).

If they need further evaluation, it's time for a stress test. So, which to pick? Speaking technically, you can combine modalities (exercise echo) but that's not routinely done. Here are the options available:

Stress Test	Indication
Exercise ECG	Normal ECG baseline Can exercise
Dobutamine Stress Echo	Abnormal ECG or Can't Exercise
Nuclear Stress	Test Abnormal Echo Previous CABG Assessing for scar

Call Cardiology
You've done MONA BASH. At some point you might call cards. They will decide if they need a cath or not. Call cards when

- ST ↑
- Troponins ↑
- Stress test is positive

Heart Failure In the Clinic – Outpatient

Categorizing & Reporting CHF.
What we actually care about is the New York Heart Association Class. It allows us to trend patients over time to see if they're improving, worsening, or staying the same.

Class	Symptoms
NYHA I	None
NYHA II	With a lot of effort (exercise)
NYHA III	With a little effort (ADLs)
NYHA IV	At Rest

Every note, every presentation, for every patient, every time must include:

Write In Note, Say In Presentation	
NYHA Class	Ranges are ok (2-3)
Systolic or Diastolic	Ace/Arb not necessary in diastolic
Ischemic or Nonischemic	Give etiology if known
Last known ejection fraction	And the date, modality (echo, nuke)

Keep track of this stuff in your note. It isn't necessary to present for every patient.

Important Information To Track	
Vitals (BP, HR)	Weight
JVD	Edema
Creatinine	K
Hgb	Current Med List

Treatment of CHF by NYHA Class
All CHF patients get a **Beta-Blocker (BB)** and an **Ace-inhibitor (ACEi)**, no matter the stage. These medications should be maxed out before others are added.

All ischemic CHF patients get an **ASA** and a **Statin**, just like CAD.

Class II **Loop diuretics** (lasix) are added when there are the symptoms of fluid.

Class III **Spironolactone** and/or **BiDil** are added when NYHA worsens or there is additional blood pressure control needed.

Class IV: Palliation or transplant. Pressors (dobutamine or milrinone) can bridge to LVAD, bridge to transplant, or destination to death. YOU will not see these patients.

EF < 35% and NOT class IV: **AICD**. Refer to EP cards for assessment for AICD and resynchronization therapy.

Non-Medication Therapy	
Diet	<2g NaCl / day
Fluid	<2L Fluid / day
Smoking	Stop Smoking (duh)
EtoH	Stop Drinking (duh)
AVOID	NSAIDs

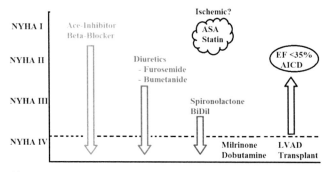

Heart Failure In the Hospital – Inpatient

Acute Decompensated Heart Failure - DX
To tread ADHF you have first categorize them to know what to do for them.

WET or DRY? They're wet if they have these things. How bad they are tells just how wet they are:

History	Physical
Dyspnea on exertion	Crackles
PND	JVD
Orthopnea	Hepatojug Reflux
Weight Gain	Peripheral Edema
Abdominal Pain	↑ BNP from baseline

WARM or COLD? Being cold is a sign of poor tissue perfusion. This is bad. Don't ignore someone who is, "too tired to talk," in the ED when they have:

History, Physical	Labs
Altered Mental Status	↓ Urine Output
Cold wrists, ankles	↑ Creatinine
Narrow Pulse Pressure	↑ LFTs
Fatigue	CI < 2.2

What about beta blockers in ADHF?
The benefit of Beta Blockers is long term. Acutely, they drop the EF and worsen ADHF. They can push someone into cold and wet. You may continue beta blockers, but do NOT start or increase BB in ADHF.

Acute Decompensated Heart Failure - TX

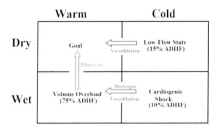

LOOPS
Furosemide	1 IV = 2 PO
Bumetanide	1 Bumex = 40 Lasix

Thiazides
Metolazone	5mg 30 min before loop
HCTZ	12.5mg, 25mg

DOSE TRIAL
- Give **IV Lasix** at **2.5x home po dose**
- **Drip = Bolus**
- Stop Lasix if the creatinine bumps.

AFTERLOAD ↓	PRELOAD ↓
Ace-inhibitors	Nitrates
CCB	Morphine
Hydralazine	Diuretics

If they are <u>hyper</u>tensive, control that BP.

If they are **cold**, it is likely from increased afterload. Reduce afterload.

If they are **wet**, reduce the preload and get rid of volume. Give them diuresis or nitrates. Use **Loops** with or without a thiazide boost (metolazone). Use only **IV diuretics** during ADHF. Gut is edematous and oral absorption is limited.

If they're **cold and wet**, called cardiogenic shock (<u>hypo</u>tensive), they need inotropic support before they get anything. Use dobutamine as it's more predictable. Because you get both vasodilation and inotropic activity, watch for DROPS in BP. You hope that by improving contractility and reducing SVR, you get a new win.

CHAPTER 6: COMMON MEDICAL PROBLEMS

Afib

Treatment for Afib with RVR
1. If they're **unstable, shock them.**
2. If they're **stable, rate control.**
   a. if No CHF --> BB or CCB
   b. If Yes CHF --> Dig... Amio
3. Consider **anticoagulation**
4. Consider **cardioversion**

Drug	Class	Notes
Diltiazem	CCB	Avoid in CHF
Metoprolol	BB	Avoid in CHF
Digoxin	Dig	First line in CHF
Amiodarone	Amio	Second Line CHF

Causes of AFib
Plumbing: Valvular lesions, CAD
Electrical: Infarction, Infiltration
Structural: CHF, Dilation
Metabolic: Holiday Heart, EtoH
Reactionary: Sepsis, PE, COPD

Cardioversion candidate (not in shock)
Usually this person has **no structural** or **electrical abnormality** (clean cath, normal EF) and is young. They'll need anticoagulation for **3 weeks prior and after** the cardioversion. Amiodarone is sometimes added to improve conversion results. **CARDIOLOGY** makes this decision.

Anticoagulation Strategies / Family Talk
Coumadin is the standard therapy. It requires an **INR check weekly for a month, monthly for a year.** The goal INR is 2-3. Coumadin for Afib **doesn't require a bridge.** Further, they can be discharged on their first dose. This anticoagulation can be reversed with Vitamin K and FFP.

Others (Pradaxa, Eliquis) are indicated for **nonvalvular Afib only.** There are no lab draws. But... these are irreversible.

Do you anticoagulate? CHADS2

C	CHF	1
H	HTN	1
A	Age > 75	1
D	Diabetes	1
S	Stroke	1
S	Stroke	1

Score	Interpretation
0	Aspirin
1	Aspirin or Coumadin or
2 +	Coumadin

Score	Interpretation
0	ASA 325
1 +	Pradaxa, Eliquis, Whatever

I want to NOT anticoagulate. HAASBLED

You just say the **risk outweighs benefits** and why (usually **risk of falls** and **discussed with family/patient**).

Objectively you can use HAASBLED

H	HTN	1
A	Abnormal Liver	1
A	Abnormal Kidney	1
S	Stroke	1
B	Bleeding	1
L	Labile INR	1
E	Elderly > 65	1
D	Drugs or EtOH	1

Score < 3	Anticoagulation safe
Score ≥ 3	Anticoagulation safety uncertain

106

COPD Exacerbation

Diagnosis and Assessment of Severity

A person in a COPD exacerbation will complain of one of two things, often presenting together:

1. Increased sputum production
2. Worsening dyspnea or exertional dyspnea

What to look for:
1. **Shortness of breath**
2. **Wheezing**
3. **Sputum production**

It would be nice to have:
1. A history of COPD
2. A history of long-term smoking
3. An **ABG** that shows CO2 retention

Look for severity:
1. Need for **Home Oxygen**
2. Known **PFTs** (don't get in-house)
3. History of **intubation** and how often
4. What their baseline meds are for COPD - the more they need at baseline the worse they are
5. Their **pH** (NOT their CO2)

Who needs to be admitted?

Anyone with a COPD exacerbation that the ED calls you for. If they're not back to baseline after a couple of duonebs, they're getting admitted.

Dispo

Rising CO2, need for BiPap or Intubation **goes to the unit.** Everyone else: **the floor.**

In COPD, **ABGs DO** play a big role. You are looking at the pCO2 and, more importantly, the pH. Some people live at a pCO2 of 80. It is the acid/base derrangement, rather than the CO2, which determines severity.

Treatment / Admit Orders

1. **Steroids**: use **IV solumedrol** if they can't tolerate po or **po prednisone** if they can.

2. **Duonebs**: albuterol/ipratropium should be given **q4h scheduled** then de-escalated. De-escalation involves first spacing them out (q6-q8), then prn, then MDI inhalers.

3. **Oxygen:** target 88-92% on pulse ox. DON'T use ABGs for oxygen assessment.

4. **Antibiotics:** Choose between **Doxycycline and Azithromycin**. People get antibiotics only if there's an increase in sputum production or purulence. They should not get what they got the last time (rotate antibiotics). Be careful of the cardiac side effects of Azithromycin (prolonged QT)

5. **Chronic Meds:** Continue Spiriva, scheduled disks, nasal sprays, and oral anti-histamines. See Common Meds section for COPD meds.

6. Pulse oximetry, either continuous or q4h.

Tips for next-leveling it

1. **Solumedrol IV** to justify inpatient
2. Duonebs **q4h** to justify inpatient
3. LOS should be ~ **3-4 days**.
4. Use **continuous nebulizers** if things aren't working.

CHAPTER 6: COMMON MEDICAL PROBLEMS

Pulmonary Embolism

Making the Diagnosis

Patients with PEs that matter will have either Tachycardia or Hypoxemia. The absence of both rules out an acute (but not chronic) Pulmonary Embolism.

Well's Criteria and Diagnostic Decisions

Well's Criteria – Calculating The Score	
ZOMFG I DONT KNOW	3
DVT	3
HR > 100	1.5
Immobilization (Leg Fx, Travel)	1.5
Surgery w/i 4 weeks	1.5
h/o DVT or PE	1.5
Hemoptysis	1
Malignancy	1

V/Q And D-Dimer Interpretation		
Score < 2	Score 2-6	Score > 6
Low Prob	Med Prob	High Prob
D-Dimer	V/Q	V/Q OK
VQ OK	Useless	

Do I Do A CT Scan?	
Score < 4 Don't Do it	Score > 4 Do it

CT PE Protocol when you want a confirmatory answer and the kidneys are good.

V/Q scan when you can't do a CT PE protocol AND the lungs are normal. This is also useful in the "rule out" category.

D-Dimer never inpatient. It's used in the outpatient setting to rule out a PE. Don't do a CT scan for a positive D-Dimer.

The 3 points on the top of the chart really mean, "I have no idea why they have shortness of breath. Just scan them to find out."

Treating a PE

Warfarin should be started the day of diagnosis. It must be **bridged with heparin**. Goal is INR 2-3. They must be on it for 5 days or when the INR is 2-3, whichever is LATER.

LMWH (Fragmin, Lovenox, Arixtra) is just as good as Unfractionated heparin, but more convenient (can be done at home,

with ↓ length of stays); they don't mandate frequent PTT checking. But, they all have a **longer half-life** and, being smaller, **can't be reversed** with protamine.

Unfractionated Heparin is the "heparin drip," a weight based dose of about 80units/kg with a protocol for adjusting the drip based on the PTT every 6 hours OR the Xa levels. It's **easily reversed** with protamine. It's indicated in **submassive PE**.

tPA is indicated in **massive PE**. There's a high bleeding risk.

Thrombectomy is considered only in Chronic Thromboembolic Pulmonary Hypertension. Specifically, in the **chronic condition** and never in the acute setting.

Vena Cava Filter. If the patient 1) has a DVT, 2) can't be anticoagulated, and 3) the next PE will kill them... then, and only then is it ok.

Diagnosis	Sxs	Strain	Shock	Tx	Dispo
Asymptomatic PE	No	No	No	LMWH	Home
Symptomatic PE	Yes	No	No	LMWH	Floor
Submassive PE	Yes	Yes	No	Heparin gtt	Unit
Massive PE	Yes	Yes	Yes	tPA	Unit
CTEPH		Thrombectomy			

108

Sepsis

1. Identify SIRS and Severity

SIRS	WBC > 12 or < 4
	HR > 90
	Temp > 38 or < 36
	RR > 20
Sepsis	SIRS + A source
Severe Sepsis	Sepsis + Hypotension responsive to fluid
Septic Shock	Sepsis + Hypotension not responsive to fluid

2. Identify Source
There are many potential sources. Everyone who has a fever gets:
- Chest X-ray
- Urinalysis, Urine Culture
- Blood Culture

Other potential sources to consider:
- SBP (paracentesis)
- Meningitis (LP)
- Cellulitis (look)
- Osteomyelitis (X-ray)

Fever Sources people miss (AEIOU)
- **A**bscess (hepatic)
- **E**ndocarditis
- **I**ndwelling Catheters
- **O**steomyelitis
- **U**TI

3. Treat Empirically

Sick as shit	Vanc + Pip/Tazo
HCAP	Vanc + Pip/Tazo
Diabetic Foot	Vanc + Pip/Tazo
CAP	Ceftri + Azithro
UTI	Ceftriaxone
Cellulitis	Vancomycin
GI source	Cipro + Metro

4. Cultures and Sensitivities
Draw cultures before giving antibiotics.

De-escalate antibiotics over time based on disease progression (defervescence of Sepsis is a good sign things are working).

Expand coverage if signs of sepsis don't resolve.

Switch to the most narrow spectrum and oral solution possible based on cultures and sensitivities.

5. Early Goal Directed therapy
a. **Fluids** - give 2-3 Liters LR
b. **Abx** - empiric
c. **Source Control** - drain abscess, remove lines
d. **Pressors** - if MAP < 65 after fluid

6. Symptoms of a UTI
For whatever reason, old people (or those with cognitive dysfunction) will present with altered mental status even from a simple UTI. It's weird but common.

7. More
Check out the Common Meds section for antibiotics

Check out the Methods section for an approach to antibiotics

Check out In The ICU for septic shock

CHAPTER 6:   COMMON MEDICAL PROBLEMS

Principles of Antibiotic Management

1. If the patient is **sick, go broad** – vanc & zosyn is ok for unit players in septic shock.
2. If the patient **isn't sick, target empirically**. Aim for **as low on the ladder** as you're able. Knowing which bugs cause the type of infections you're dealing with are crucial.
3. Double cover pseudomonas
4. Penicillins have 1% cross-reactivity with cephalosporins. They are ok to give to someone with a penicillin allergy EXCEPT in anaphylaxis.
5. Use **cultures and sensitivities** to get **oral** and **targeted therapy**
6. See Common Meds – Antibiotics for **empiric coverage by diagnosis**

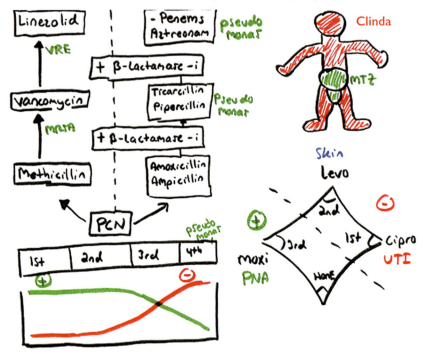

Classes:

1. Fluoroquinolones: you have to go past first base to get to third base. High generation FQs retain the previous generation, but gain more gram positive coverage.
2. Anaerobes: **Metronidazole** for the gut and vagina, **Clindamycin** for everywhere else.
3. Cephalosporins:
    - 1st Generations cover skin flora, gram positives
    - 3rd Generations cover Gram negatives and positives (Ceftriaxone)
    - 4th Generations cover pseudomonas (**Cefepime**)

Pneumonia

Making the Diagnosis
Pneumonia has a very simple diagnosis
1. Fever
2. Cough
3. X-ray showing consolidation

Don't be fooled by "infiltrate" on an X-ray. If the clinical picture doesn't fit, don't call it pneumonia.

Identifying an Organism
1. Do get blood cultures
2. DON'T get sputum cultures (intubated bronchs are different)
3. Do get FLU swab during FLU season

Generally, the culture doesn't change management, antibiotic choice, or duration. The utility of sputum sample is limited by normal respiratory flora.

Types of Pneumonia
Stop saying typical or atypical. Nothing in the labs, physical, or presentation can separate the potential organism. The etiology doesn't matter (sort of). Here's what DOES matter.

Type	What Makes It That Type
CAP	No association with healthcare
HCAP	Hospital, NH, HD w/i 90 days
HAP	Pna 2 days after admission
VAP	Pneumonia on a ventilator

Core Measures
1. Cultures before abx
2. Antibiotics within 6 hours
3. Oxygen assessment (Spo2, ABG)
4. Smoking cessation
5. Vaccines

Determining Severity and Disposition
ED uses CURB-65 (admit or no)
ICU uses SMARTCOP (pressors)
YOU use the Pneumonia Severity Index

	Pneumonia Severity Index	
	Factor	Pts
	Age	Starting #
	Female	-10
History	Nursing Home	+10
	Cancer	+30
	Liver Disease	+20
	CHF	+10
	CVA	+10
	CKD	+10
Physical	AMS	+20
	RR > 29	+20
	SYS BP < 90	+20
	Temp <35 or > 40	+15
	HR > 124	+10
	pH <7.35	+30
Labs	BUN > 29	+20
	Sodium < 130	+20
	Glucose > 250	+10
	Hct < 30%	+10
	PaO2 < 60	+10
	Effusion	+10

Start with the age. Then add values as you find them. The total puts them in a class.

Class	Points	Action
I	0	Ambulatory Treatment
II	<70	Ambulatory Treatment
III	71-90	Admit to floor, IV abx
IV	91-130	Admit to floor, IV abx
V	>130	Admit to ICU, IV abx

Type	Treatment (With Alternates)
CAP	Azithro-only for ambulatory pts
CAP	Ceftriaxone and Azithro (Moxifloxacin)
HAP	Vancomycin and Zosyn
VAP	(Linezolid) (Meropenem)
HCAP	

CHAPTER 6: COMMON MEDICAL PROBLEMS

Electrolytes - Sodium

Sodium concentrations have nothing to do with salt. Instead, they're associated with free water. In other words, Sodium is a marker for water.

High Sodium = too little water
Low sodium = too much water

Hypernatremia
Hypernatremia means there's a **free water deficit**. Thus, the goal is to give free water.
1. Replace **volume deficit** with **large volume resuscitation** (either LR or NS), knowing that there are 154mEq of sodium in each. Which means, if the sodium concentration is LESS than 154, you might INCREASE it.
2. Replace **free water deficit**.
Use an online calculator to determine the free water deficit. Doing it by hand is mentally draining and lends itself to mistakes. Take the RATE and a FLUID

Method	When To Use	Comments
Oral Water	Best	No restriction
NG Tube free water flushes	Best	If NPO or can't tolerate oral
D5W	Best IV option	Most Dilute IV fluid
1/2NS	Other IV option	Higher rates than D5W
D5 1/2NS	Hypertonic	Will HURT. NOT THIS

3. Check to assure the corrections aren't too fast. Get **BMPs** every 4 hours initially, then twice daily. The goal is 2mEq every q4h BMP, or a rate of 0.25mEq / **hour**.

Some exceptions apply

Hyponatremia
Hyponatremia is a whole hell of a lot harder than hyper. There are many things to consider, and the discussion is quite lengthy. Check out the Na content on how to actually work up a patient with low sodium.

1. Replace the **solute deficit**
Use an online calculator to determine the free water deficit. Doing it by hand is mentally draining and lends itself to mistakes. Take the RATE and a FLUID

What You Get	Why
Serum Osms	Assure it's real
Urine Osms	ADH Surrogate
Urine Sodium	Aldosterone Surrogate

Value	What It Means
Serum Osm < 280	Truly hypotonic
Urine Osms >300	ADH off
Urine Na > 20	Aldosterone Off
Urine Na < 10	Aldosterone ON

What You Do	Why
3% NaCl (Hypertonic)	Na < 110, Coma, Seizures
Lasix	Volume Overloaded
Bolus LR or 0.9% NaCl	Volume Deplete
Volume restrict	Euvolemic

Electrolytes - Potassium

Potassium (K) is tightly regulated; it should be between 4.0 and 5.0.

Hypokalemia
Hypokalemia should be repleted. The goal is to provide it orally when able, IV only if unable.

Oral	Elixir
Oral	Tab
Intravenous	IV Bag

Current K	K Required To Move 0.1
3.0 - 4.0	10mEq
2.5-3.0	15mEq
2.0-2.5	20mEq

A common way to give potassium is to give 40mEq at one time. This is what's done when they're close (almost 4) and you want to assure they stay there.

But, repleting K when it's actually low is more challenging. You can do **40mEq po with each meal** (total of 120mEq), while **backing it up with IV KCL** concurrently.

KCL can be administered **10mEq/hr** through a **peripheral IV** because it burns. It will go faster (**20mEq/hr**) through a **central line**.

DON'T WAIT to start repleting.
DON'T BE SHY on the amount they need.

YOU WILL get a call from pharmacy. Explain to them 1) going from 3.0 to 4.0 requires 100mEq, and 2) most of the time you're giving something that depletes K further (IV fluids, Lasix).

Replete **magnesium before or at the same time as K**. Mag is needed to keep K.

Potassium outside the normal ranges causes cardiac arrhythmias and death.

Hyperkalemia
There are two pathways of Hyperkalemia:

1. Hey, their potassium is high, but there aren't ECG changes. **Reduce total body potassium.**

2. The potassium is high and, CRAP! ECG CHANGES! **Stabilize, Temporize, AND reduce total body potassium!**

The hinge point is whether or not there are **peaked T-waves** or **Widened QRS** associated with the high K.

Drug	Does
IV Calcium	Stabilize
Beta Agonists	Temporize
Sodium Bicarb	Temporize
Insulin + D50	Temporize
Lasix	↓ Total Body K
Kayexalate (stool)	↓ Total Body K
Dialysis	↓ Total Body K

Any instance of hyperkalemia is going to get some treatment to bring the total body K down.

Only instances of hyperkalemia with ECG changes get IV Calcium. If they do, they must also get a temporizing agent and an agent to drop total body K. **IV calcium lasts minutes** and stabilizes the cardiac myocytes to prevent sine-wave arrest. The **temporizing agents** shift potassium into cells, but that shift is transient. Only **total body K reducers** actually save the patient in the long run.

CHAPTER 6: COMMON MEDICAL PROBLEMS

Cirrhosis

Once a patient has cirrhosis it's forever... there's no going back. But having cirrhosis doesn't matter until they **decompensate**. Decompensation isn't like CHF. It's not an acute exacerbation, but rather a chronic decompensation. You are decompensated if you have any one of: **ascites, varices,** or **encephalopathy**.

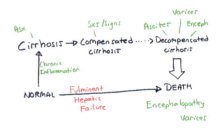

1. Ascites
Low Oncotic Pressure from low albumin. This causes fluid to leak out of the portal system. **Albumin infusions don't help**, they are too short lived. Albumin infusions DO prevent hypotension after a large volume paracentesis, but not in chronic management.

Increased hydrostatic pressure from portal hypertension doubles the effect of low oncotic pressure. More fluid in the abdomen.

Activation of the renin-angio-aldo axis causes resorption of fluid. That fluid ends up in vasodilated splanchnic vessels, worsening ascites.

Ascites is treated with a **low-volume** low salt **diet** and **diuretics**. It's not uncommon to see **Furosemide and Spironolactone used** in amazingly high doses to treat ascites.

TIPS procedure is used only for when portal hypertension causes fatal conditions (Varices) as a bridge to transplant. A TIPS procedure will cause hepatic encephalopathy.

If no SBP, you can do a **large-volume paracentesis** for relief of their ascites (temporarily). Give 25g IV Albumin following a therapeutic paracentesis.

Things that cause put your AST and ALT into the thousands cause Fulminant Hepatic Failure:
1. Acetaminophen
2. Afla Toxin
3. Acute Viral Hepatitis
4. Autoimmune Hepatitis
5. Budd-Chiari

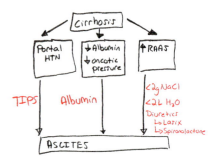

6. Shock Liver

Repeated therapeutic paracenteses may be needed as the fluid is just going to reaccumulate

114

Cirrhosis

2. SBP
Spontaneous Bacterial Peritonitis kills cirrhotics. Anyone with ascites gets a **diagnostic paracentesis** if it's their first presentation OR if they're coming in for a worsening of their condition.

ALL admits get a diagnostic tap. Rule out SBP in every cirrhotic-with-ascites admit.

If >**250 neutrophils**, you have made the diagnosis, and you treat with **ceftriaxone**.

Prophylaxis is done with **Cipro** if you've ever had SBP or if the Total Protein is < 1.0

3. Diagnosing Ascites - SAAG
The **Serum Ascites Albumin Gradient** (serum albumin – ascites albumin) tells the likely etiology.

A SAAG of ≥ 1.1 is portal hypertension related. It's most likely cirrhosis.

A SAAG of < 1.1 is oncotic related. It's likely cancer or an infection.

4. Esophageal Varices
Esophageal varices are the only porto-caval shunts that matter. Screen cirrhotics with EGD to see if they have one.

In outpatient, give **nadolol** or **propranolol** to keep the portal pressures low and the varices small.

In inpatient, give **IV PPI, IV ceftriaxone** (SBP prophylaxis), and **octreotide**.

EGD is required to clip the varices. Do it within 6 hours. **HOLD BETA BLOCKERS DURING ANY ACUTE BLEED**

Transfuse to a hemoglobin of 7.

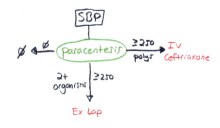

↑Parterial	↓σ_{int} or K
Portal HTN Related	Non-Portal HTN Related
SAAG ≥ 1.1	SAAG < 1.1
Cirrhosis	**Cancer** **Peritoneal TB**
R-sided CHF Budd-Chiari Portal/Splenic Thrombosis Schistosomiasis	Nephrotic Syndrome Protein-Losing Enteropathy Post-Op Lymphatic Leak Bowel Obstruction

115

4. Hepatic Encephalopathy

Hepatic encephalopathy comes from elevated ammonium in the brain.

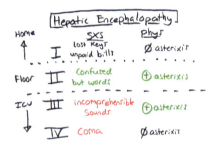

The level of ammonia in the blood doesn't correlate with the level of ammonium in the brain. **Stop checking ammonia levels**; do a physical exam instead.

The only way to get the ammonia out of the body is through stool. Achieve that with lactulose.

Asterixis is the loss of tone and quickly regaining it. You don't have to see hand-flapping. Eye-closing, toe-pushing, and finger-squeezing all work.

Additive therapies are **rifaximin** and **zinc**. Grade on severity and dispo them appropriately. See chart.

5. Acute Exacerbation

Fluid: Albumin bolus

If **MELD ↑**, **Cr ↑**, or they come in with **Altered Mental Status** assume there is a problem with **Fluid, Infection**, or **Bleed**.

Infection: Panculture, Give Antibiotics

Bleed: H/H, transfusion, EGD for varices

Cirrhotics are fragile. In the acute setting, DO MORE than less. Even if it seems like "just medication noncompliance" do it all. If you don't, you're going to kill someone. DO MORE. NOT LESS

MELD: Calculated by INR, T. bili, Cr. The higher the MELD, the sicker they are.

– Transplant at 15
– Cancer gives a 22
– Transplant happens at 32
– Death occurs at 40

Cirrhotics may not present with sepsis. In fact, **their SIRS criteria is a rise in the MELD**.

Document a MELD every office visit, every day in the hospital, every admit and every discharge.

Don't get tricked. Cirrhotics are sick at baseline. Their therapeutic window is small; they die fast.

CIRRHOSIS

6. Hepato-Renal Syndrome
This is a death sentence. Do everything possible to prove it isn't this. Start with Fluid, Infection, and Bleed.

Give Albumin. 25g IV q8 day 1 and day 3. Give **octreotide** and **midodrine**.

Treat infections. Panculture, give broad spectrum antibiotics. Don't forget SBP. Always tap a cirrhotic coming into the hospital (if there is an ascites, of course).

Bleed. Watch the H/H. Replace as needed.

Urine Sodium will show prerenal.

If you diagnose HRS Type I don't do dialysis. Don't treat. If they can't be transplanted, it's over – they're dead. If you can transplant, get them to a transplant center. Dialysis will prolong suffering.

7. Hepato-Pulmonary Syndrome
Vasodilation is the pathophysiology of cirrhosis. It makes sense that this might happen in the lungs, too. The problem with this condition is that the red blood cells may not actually get up against the capillary wall, which **impairs oxygen delivery**. Diagnose with a **Bubble Study** (3-6 beats). Look for **platypnea** (the opposite of orthopnea).

8. Portopulmonary Hypertension
People with cirrhosis can get pulmonary hypertension, even though we just learned about the opposite problem. Get an Echo and **right heart cath** before every transplant (you'll get a left heart cath also). The problem stems from releasing all that portal pressure into the vena cava. If there's pulmonary hypertension, it overloads the RV, backing up fluid into the liver, resulting in loss of the transplanted liver.

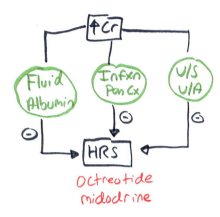

HRS-Type I
Double the creatinine
Half the creatinine clearance

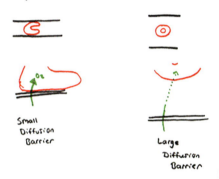

Happens within 2 weeks

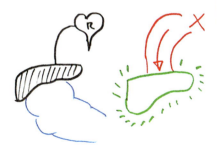

9. Transplant

The sicker the liver (the higher the MELD) the more likely the patient is to get one. There must be an HLA match, of course, but if/when there is the highest need gets it.

10. Hepatocellular Carcinoma

Screening is done with **AFP** and **Ultrasound**. It can be diagnosed without a biopsy. How frequently you do this, however, is dependent on the underlying patient.

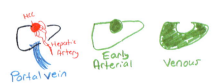

Diagnosis is made with the **triple phase CT** (early arterial, late arterial, venous). HCC is fed by the hepatic artery. It lights up in the arterial phase, but not in the venous phase. The effect is called **washout**. The liver gets most of its blood from the portal vein. It lights up during venous, but not arterial phase.

Cancer present (lights up) during arterial phase because it's fed by hepatic artery while the liver does not light up (not filled in) because it receives portal blood.

Liver present during venous phase while the cancer is not.

Treatment is based on the MILAN criteria. Remember 3 and 3, 1 and 5. MILAN is less than 3 lesions as long as each are less than 3cm, or any one lesion that is less than 5cm. Don't transplant if they're "outside MILAN." Instead, get them inside Milan using RFA (Radiofrequency Ablation) or TACE.

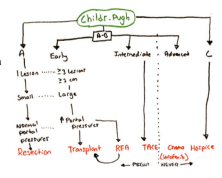

If you can't get them close, use **palliative Sorafenib**. Or, simply put them into **Hospice** if their Childs-Pugh score is too bad. While not designed for the MELD, the same idea predominates: too sick for a transplant means sick enough for hospice.

GI Bleed

GI Bleeds can be scary. They kill people. The blood just keeps coming and there's no way to tamponade it.

Having an advanced organizer for the causes of GI bleed is useful, but it really doesn't matter because YOUR steps will almost always be the same.

Hematemesis is the only reliable finding. It means there **must be an upper GI bleed source**.

While **melena** is suggestive of upper and **hematochezia** is suggestive of lower, it could be misleading. Bright red blood per rectum could be a brisk upper, fast middle, or just lower GI bleed. Be careful when using reasoning to decide upper from lower.

Regardless, you'll **do the same five things for every GI bleeder**. Will it be too much sometimes? Sure. But it may just save someone's life. It's worth it. See the table.

To decide who needs the **ICU** do one test: **orthostatics**. If the blood pressure is ever low (either without orthostatics or if orthostatics are positive) they go to the unit.

You won't fix a GI bleed. GI does that with a scope. You'll **keep them alive**. Give them **blood and fluids**. If more than 3 units of PRBC are needed, give **3 pRBC** to **1 FFP** to **1 6-pack platelets** and monitor Ca.

Short, stubby, thick lines are best (large bore peripherals). TLC lines, while three 18G lines, are too long (and limit the rate of transfusion). Use a Cordis if central access is needed. Or, get a TLC for the NON-blood infusions

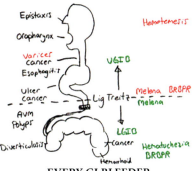

EVERY GI BLEEDER

2 Large Bore IVs (18G or bigger)
IV Fluid bolus (2L LR)
Type and Cross, transfuse as needed
IV Protonix
GI Consult

IF CIRRHOTIC, ADD

IV ceftriaxone
IV Octreotide

WHO GOES TO THE UNIT

Orthostatics are positive → ICU
Frankly hypotensive → ICU
Ongoing obvious hemorrhage → ICU
Variceal Bleeder → ICU

PRESSOR OF CHOICE FOR GI BLEED

Blood. Or Fluid. But Blood.

PRINCIPLES OF LINE MANAGEMENT

2 Short, 18G lines >> One Triple Lumen
Central access = Cordis
Length of catheter limits transfusion rates more than the caliber

CHAPTER 6: COMMON MEDICAL PROBLEMS

Approach to LFTs

These LFT sticks are different than what you'll find in most printed material. This way makes more sense. You will see why.

The things listed in black (TP, Albumin, AST, ALT) are markers of liver function. They're **hepatocellular**. The Total Protein and Albumin represent **chronic synthetic function** (along with INR), while the AST and ALT represent **acute hepatocellular injury**.

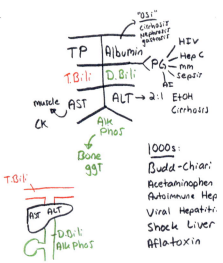

The things listed in green (Direct Bili, Alk Phos) are markers of biliary function. They're going to be elevated in **obstructive** or post-hepatic pathologies.

The thing listed in red (T. Bili) can go up with the D. Bili or the Indirect Bilirubin. If only the bili is elevated, chances are it's simply **hemolysis** within the blood. The rate limiting step of bilirubin metabolism is the conversion of unconjugated (blood) to conjugated (biliary tree) bilirubin.

The difference between the Total Protein and the Albumin is the **protein gap**. If it's **greater than 4** you have immunoglobulins. Think **HIV, Hep C** and **Multiple Myeloma**. The game doesn't end there, but it often gets you the answer.

GGT comes from the biliary tree, while Alk Phos comes from both **bone and the biliary tree**. GGT will confirm an elevated ALP is from the biliary system.

AST is in muscle also. A **CK** can separate muscle from liver (CK elevated in muscle breakdown like rhabdo).

An **AST:ALT ratio > 2:1** is suggestive of both **alcoholic hepatitis** and **cirrhosis**.

Only a few things push the **AST or ALT** into the **4 digit range**. That list is 6 items strong.

- Shock
- Acute Viral Hepatitis (A, B)
- Autoimmune Hepatitis
- Acetaminophen
- Aflatoxin
- Budd-Chiari

Finally, a **low albumin** is associated with the "osi." A patient either loses protein through urine (**nephrosis**, nephrotic syndrome), can't build albumin (**cirrhosis**) or can't absorb it (**gastrosis, protein malnutrition**.)

INPATIENT DIABETES

Inpatient Diabetes

Inpatient diabetes management is really easy. Like NIKE, just do it.

STOP ALL ORAL MEDICATIONS.

First, figure out the **total daily insulin**. It'll either be **0.5U/kg** (1/2 body weight) or **0.3 U/kg** (1/3 body weight).

Ok. So the total daily insulin's been calculated. Do this the right way. Since the person is in house, it's easy to do (the nurse injects and checks sugars, not the patient).

½ **Total Daily Insulin** is given **basal qHs.**

½ **Total Daily Insulin** is given **bolus**, divided between three meals, **qAc.**

Then add the **supplemental sliding scale** on top of what was calculated. Make sure the sliding scale insulin type is **THE SAME TYPE AS THE BOLUS (qAC) INSULIN.**

Multiple steps, actually very easy.

Then, each day take the total sliding scale given and divide it up - ½ to basal, ½ to bolus. Essentially, just add it to the total daily insulin and divide it up like you did above.

But hey, what if they go NPO?
They're on qAc and qHs; they need the basal insulin all the time. They don't need the prandial insulin unless they eat. But they aren't eating. So you won't check, you won't give insulin, and they won't eat. Boom.

If they go for prolonged periods of NPO, then sure, do a supplemental without scheduled.

Total Daily Insulin			
0.5 Units /Kg		**0.3 Units / Kg**	
Cr <1.5	And	Cr > 1.5	Or
Age <70	And	Age > 70	Or
bG > 180		bG < 180	

Long Acting (Basal)	Short Acting (Prandial)
Lantus	Novolog
Levemir	Humalog

Don't Use These Inpatient	
Novolin 70/30	Novolin 50/50
Humalin 70/30	Humanlin 50/50
NPH	

Sliding Scale	
bG	**Action**
<70	Hypoglycemia
70-150	No Sliding Scale
151-200	1 Units
201-250	2 Units
251-300	3 Units
301-350	4 Units
350+	5 Units

Sliding scale insulin = prandial insulin

An Example:
100kg dude. He's 50. His creatinine is 0.9
TDI = 50% Body weight = 50 Units

Basal = 50% TDI = 25 Units qHs
Bolus = 50% TDI = 25 units

Bolus / 3 meals = 8 units qAc

His regimen is 25 qHs, 8 qAc

COMMON PROBS

CHAPTER 6:   COMMON MEDICAL PROBLEMS

Diabetic Ketoacidosis

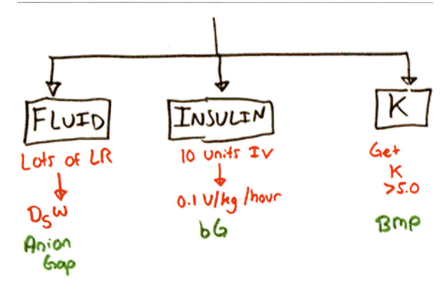

Diagnosing DKA isn't hard; they'll have **D K** and **A**. D is for **Diabetes**, usually an elevated sugar (very few conditions can have a normal or not-very-elevated sugar and be in DKA). They'll also have **Ketones** (in the urine or in the blood, either is fine). Finally there'll be **Acidosis**.

That means a **BMP**, a **urinalysis**, and an **ABG** are needed.

These people are **volume down** (unless they're ESRD) as glucose is the most potent diuretic there is. They're dehydrated, sick, and regardless of how long they've been in DKA, should be considered critical.

While mild DKA can be managed on the floor, what I want you to see is, "If DKA, go to unit." That way less time is spent thinking about how severe they are and more time is used actually giving them fluid and insulin (following the **three-pronged approach** to DKA).

DIABETIC KETOACIDOSIS

Treatment -- open UpToDate on your computer and follow the algorithm.

1. Fluid: Fluid first.
   a. Start with **lactated ringers**. Bolus 2 liters, then set a rate that's fast (~250cc/hr).
   b. If bG < 250 and gap not closed, change to **D5½NS**. They'll need the sugar for the insulin to work on. Remember, it's the gap you care about, not the glucose.

2. Insulin:
   a. Give **10 units rapid insulin** bolus (Novolog, Humalog, Regular insulin).
   b. Begin **0.1 Unit / Kg insulin drip**.
   c. Titrate the insulin drip so that the sugar decreases by 75/hour.
   d. As the gap closes bridge with **SubQ long acting insulin** (NPH, Lantus, Levemir).
   e. Wean off insulin drip (don't stop until the gap remains closed).

3. Potassium: Insulin shifts K into cells. Replete potassium before giving insulin.
   a. If K > 5.0 do nothing.
   b. If K 3.5-5.0 start 10Eq/hour with fluids and insulin.
   c. If **K < 3.5 hold insulin** and give both oral and IV Potassium. DON'T hold fluids.

4. Anion Gap:
   a. Follow q4h.
   b. Track **Potassium** and replete as needed (give Mag first).
   c. Track the **Anion Gap**, which is the only way to know the DKA is resolved.

From there, investigate the cause of DKA. The common ones are non-compliance, infection, trauma, infarction, and illicit drug use. Then, initiate the appropriate work-up for precipitating events (culture, CXR, EKG, cardiac enzymes).

CHAPTER 6: COMMON MEDICAL PROBLEMS

Outpatient Diabetes

Outpatient diabetes is actually far harder than inpatient. There are many more options and this and that treatment must be weighted.

But, if you follow these simple rules (ignore pharma and TV) you'll be fine.

Someone has diabetes.

Start with metformin. Metformin is contraindicated in renal disease and CHF.

If more coverage is needed **add sulfonylurea**.

TZDs are still good drugs. But, no one will let you use them because of 1-800-bad-drug. So they're out.

If you can't use metformin, **any other oral medication** can be picked.

Once on two oral drugs, that's it. If more coverage is still needed, it's time to **start insulin**.

Begin with **long acting insulin, 0.1 Units / kg basal** at night.

Have the patient check their **fasting morning sugar** and titrate up, slowly, until the fasting blood glucose is at goal.

Then move onto individual meals with **short acting insulin** - one meal at a time.

However, there are options. You could instead do **idiot insulin**. That's **bid intermediate acting** insulin. It requires no glucose checks.

Follow Total Daily Insulin from inpatient diabetes. Only do 2/3 AM and 1/3 PM. The insulin type is the same.

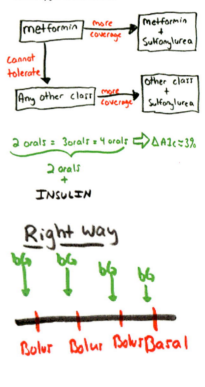

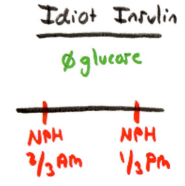

Stroke

BP Goals In Stroke (24 Hours)	
Stroke, tPA	BP Goal < 180 / <105
Stroke, no TPA	BP Goal < 220 / < 120
Hemorrhagic	MAP < 110

Anti-Platelet	
Aspirin 325	First Day, ED med
Aspirin 81	Stroke
Aggrenox	Stroke on ASA
Plavix 75	Can't have aspirin
Plavix 75 + ASA 81	New hotness

Anticoagulation	
Coumadin	For Afib
NOAC	no bridge required

tPA

Indications
<4.5 hours onset
<3 if diabetic

Contraindications
Brain Bleed… ever
Head trauma
Brain Cancer, AVM
Seizure with CVA
INR > 1.7, Plt <100
Heparin within 48h

Relative Contraindications
Trauma w/i 2 weeks
GI Bleed w/i 2 weeks
Surgery w/i 2 weeks
Pericarditis
CPR

The Work-Up

ECG*	Afib
Echo*	Clot
Ultrasound*	Carotid Stenosis
MRI	Diagnosis
CTA or MRA	Vasculitis

Every stroke, every TIA gets this

DVT Prophylaxis	
Stroke tPA	After 24 hours
Stroke, no tPA	Immediately
Hemorrhagic	24 hours after hematoma stabalizes

Code FAST

ECG	
Blood Glucose	Correct hypo
Neuro Exam	Is there a deficit
Non-Con CT	Blood or no Blood

Hemorrhagic Stroke

Reverse anticoagulation
MAP < 110
Call neurosurgery
Serial Non-Con CT

Every Stroke patient should meet these...

Core Measures

PT Eval and treat
OT eval and treat
ST eval for swallow study (npo until done)
Anti-platelet by day 2
CT or MRI of brain
Carotid Ultrasound and Echo
Statin

Risk Factor Management

HTN	<140 / < 90
DM	A1c < 7.0
Smoking	Cessation
Cholesterol	High potency statin
Plaques	Anti-platelet

Who Goes To The Unit

Strokes that get tPA
Strokes that are worsening
Hemorrhagic Strokes
Strokes that require BP drips
All for q1h neurochecks.

Intern Notes

There are some things that you won't see that often.

Some things that don't need their own page

but

things that are important enough to be written down with quick access

This is also the place where you get to write your own notes.

Thus, lots of white space.

CHAPTER 7: INTERN NOTES

Cardiology

Coronary Artery Disease

See Common Medical Problems

1. Diamond Classification
   a. Exertional
   b. Left sided, substernal
   c. Relieved with nitro
2. Associated Symptoms
   a. (Pre)Syncope
   b. Diaphoresis
   c. Dyspnea
3. Risk Factors
   a. HTN
   b. DM
   c. HLD
   d. Obesity
   e. Smoking
4. Diagnosis
   a. ECG changes, 12-lead q6H → STEMI
   b. Troponins q6 H → NSTEMI (above 1.0 "counts")
   c. Stress test
   d. Cath
5. Treatment
   a. Every patient: ASA, Statin, BB, Ace-inhibitor
   b. Every true MI: <u>M</u>orphine, <u>O</u>xygen, <u>N</u>itrates, <u>A</u>spirin, <u>B</u>eta-<u>B</u>locker, <u>A</u>ce-I, <u>S</u>tatin, <u>H</u>eparin
      i. Full dose Lovenox or Heparin gtt
      ii. Plavix load 300mg x1 then 75 daily
   c. Call cards

128

CARDIOLOGY

Congestive Heart Failure

See common medical problems

1. Ischemic or nonischemic
   a. Nuclear Stress or Left Heart Cath
2. Systolic or Diastolic ("preserved ejection fraction")
   a. Everything I tell you is known for Systolic, presumed for diastolic
   b. Heart failure "counts" when the EF is < 40%
3. Diagnosis
   a. BNP - <200 = no CHF, >500 = yes CHF, in between = ?
   b. Echo
      i. EF ↓ is Systolic CHF
      ii. E/A ↓ is Diastolic CHF (some cardiologist will say how bad)
4. Treatment
   a. Ischemic = ASA and Statin
   b. Everyone = Ace-I, Beta Blocker
   c. Symptomatic = furosemide
   d. Worsening = spironolactone or isosorbide-dinitrate / hydralazine
5. CHF exacerbations
   a. IV furosemide > PO furosemide
   b. Lasix = Bumex, no matter what someone tells you
   c. Consider inotropes (Dobutamine)

Pericardial Disease

1. <u>Pericarditis</u>
   An inflammation of the sack around the heart. It can be caused by anything, but
   uremia, viral, and **post-MI** are common. Diagnose with **PR-segment depression**
   or **diffuse-ST-segment elevation**. Treat with **NSAIDs.** Steroids are ok, especially if
   NSAIDs can't be given, but avoid in most cases (causes rebound).
2. <u>Pericardial effusion</u>
   Fluid around the heart. This is seen as dark stuff (fluid) in between the grey thing
   that is moving (the heart) and the bright white thing (the pericardium). Usually, it
   doesn't matter. If there's **tamponade** (clinical diagnosis not an echocardiographic
   one), emergent therapy is needed. If not, you have time. Refractory effusions get
   pericardial window (CT surgery). Otherwise, just try diuresis.
      - Pericardiocentesis = Tamponade
      - Pericardial Window = Recurrent or Refractory
      - Pericardectomy = Constrictive Pericarditis (this is never the diagnosis)
      - Diuresis = what you do for the pleural effusion

NOTES

CHAPTER 7: INTERN NOTES

Hypertension

JNC-7 is still the way to go

	SYS	DIA	Treatment
Normal	<120	<80	Lifestyle
Pre-Htn	120-140	80-90	Lifestyle
Stage I	≥ 140	> 90	HCTZ
Stage II	≥ 160	> 100	Comorbidities
Urgency	≥ 180	> 110	PO meds
Emergency	End-Organ Damage		IV meds

Renal Disease = Ace-I
Heart Disease = Ace-I, Beta-Blocker
Diabetes = Ace-I
Stroke = Ace-I

JNC-8 is a little different

1. BP goal is 150/90
   a. Don't try so hard for numbers. Go as low as the person will tolerate going without symptoms. Weigh risk and benefit of increasing or adding meds
2. Don't use Beta-blockers for blood pressure control
3. HTN is racist, so black people get treated differently than white people (REALLY!?)
4. Calcium Channel Blockers → Ace-I → Diuretics

Cholesterol

If they have vascular disease (CAD, PVD, CVA, Diabetes) → high potency statin
          Rosuvastatin 40   Atorvastatin 80
If they have risk factors for vascular disease → medium potency statin
          Rosuvastatin 20   Atorvastatin 40

Don't check LFTs
Don't check cholesterol (no goal) except to confirm compliance

If they have a problem, go low-potency or lower the dose.
          Pravastatin   Lovastatin   Simvastatin

Pulmonary

Asthma

1. **Chronic**
    Adults can have asthma. But if they do, they almost always had it as a child. You won't have to worry about diagnosing asthma, but you will have to manage it. Just know that it's a **reversible obstructive lung disease** that's diagnosed with **PFTs** showing **reversibility** (either methacholine induction or bronchodilator relief).

The goal is also to get patients to stop smoking and remove allergens (pets, dust, carpet, pillows) to reduce symptoms. Controlling allergies will also help. If there's a particular trigger, avoid it.

Stage	Daytime Sxs	Nocturnal Sxs	PFTs	Medications
Stage I	< 2 / week	< 2 /month	100%	SABA
Stage II	< 1 / day	< 1 / week	80%	Add ICS
Stage III	≥ 1 / day	> 1 / week	60-80%	Add ↑ dose ICS
Stage IV	≥ 1 / day	Frequent	≤ 60%	Add LABA
Stage V		Refractory		Add Steroids

2. **Exacerbations**
    Monitor the patient's response using **Peak Flows, O2 Sats** and **air movement**. Everyone gets steroids (IV Methylprednisolone and a prednisone taper to prevent rebound) and DuoNebs. Things like racemic epinephrine, terbutaline, or magnesium can also be used for rescue therapies (these latter three are in the unit). **DON'T USE BIPAP** in asthma. If they need ventilatory support, just intubate. The more times someone's been intubated the greater the likelihood that they'll need intubation this time.

Pleural Effusions

Try diuresis if they have heart failure. If they get smaller, leave them alone. If they don't, work them up. Use an **ultrasound at bedside** to decide if you can tap or not. Don't tap loculated effusions (CT surgery will) or small effusions (no one does).

Light's Criteria: if any ONE of these is met, it's Exudate, **NONE = Transudate**
1. Fluid Total Protein : Serum Total Protein > 0.5
2. Fluid LDH : Serum LDH > 0.6
3. Pleural effusion LDH > 2/3 upper limit of normal

Exudate: TB, PE, Cancer
Transudate: CHF, Cirrhosis, Nephrosis

CHAPTER 7: INTERN NOTES

COPD

1. Chronic
   a. SABA
   b. Tiotropium + SABA
   c. LABA
   d. LABA + ICS
   e. Tiotropium + SABA + ICS/LABA + PDE-4-i
   f. Add oral Steroids
2. Exacerbations
   a. IV Methylprednisolone day 0 in ED (inpatient criteria) then PO steroids
   b. Duonebs q4H scheduled… q4h prn… MDIs q4h prn as they get better
   c. Continue home inhalers (Tiotroprium, Advair, Pulmicort, whatever)
   d. SpO2 titrated to 88-92%
   e. Antibiotics for people with productive sputum or sirs
      i. Azithro or Doxy, rotate them (no pneumonia)
      ii. Ceftriaxone and Azithro (yes pneumonia)
3. Bridging PAP to Tube
   a. BiPap works great for COPD
4. Intubation
   a. CO2 rising
   b. Tiring out
   c. "anticipated need for intubation"
5. Followup
   a. Oxygen requirements are – SpO2 < 88%, PaO2 < 55
   b. Smoking Cessation
   c. Pulmonary Rehab

DVT PE

Use the **Well's Criteria** to decide what to do. **D-Dimer** when there's no chance it's a PE - that helps confirm your lack of suspicion. **V/Q scan** if their lungs are good or their creatinine is bad. **CT scan** if their lungs are bad (also the diagnostic step of choice)

Treat based on severity

1. Asymptomatic PE – Lovenox to Coumadin bridge, send home from ED
2. Symptomatic PE – Lovenox to Coumadin bridge, observe on floor
3. Submassive PE – heparin drip to Coumadin bridge, monitor in unit
4. Massive PE – tPA, admit to unit

132

PULMONARY

High Res Vs CT Scan with IV Contrast

High Resolution CT scans have thin cuts. The **interstitium** can be seen really well (in high resolution). But, there are few cuts - you may miss large masses. Get this for interstitial lung disease.

CT Scan with IV contrast takes big cuts. There's very poor resolution, but you catch **large masses** and **blood vessels**. Do this for **parenchymal disease**.

Pulmonary Nodules And Lung Cancer
Cancers

Cancer	Path	Location	Paraneoplastic	Treatment
Small Cell	Smoking	Sentral	ADH ACTH	Chemo and Radiation
Squamous Cell	Smoking	Sentral	PTH-rp	
Adenocarcinoma	Asbestos	Peripheral		
Carcinoid	-	-	Serotinin	5-HIAA Urine

Is it cancer?

1. Screening
   a. Smoking, Age > 55, smoked in last 15 → High Res CT
2. Pulmonary Nodules
   a. Assess risk of patient (smoker, occupational exposure)
   b. Assess risk of nodule (non-calcified, large, spiculated nodes)
   c. Follow as closely as q3months or as leniently as q1 year
   d. Stop after stability for 2 years

Who to call to make the diagnosis

Pulmonary – endobronchial biopsy, ultrasound

IR – CT guided biopsy

CT surgery – VATS, Surgery

You – Pleural Effusion, Tap

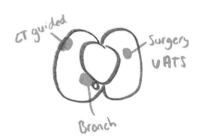

The thing to the right is a CT scan cross section showing where things are located to what you get to do it.

CHAPTER 7: INTERN NOTES

Renal Nephrology Kidney

Hypokalemia

1. Replacement is crucial
   a. **Magnesium** must be replaced first or at the same time
   b. How much given is dependent on what it is right now

K Level	mEq To Move K 0.1
3.0-4.0	10
2.5-3.0	15
2.0-2.5	20

2. Determining why it's low is sort of important
   a. GI causes: diarrhea
   b. Renal causes:
      i. Increased distal flow: diuretics OR large volume IV fluids
      ii. Increased Aldosterone: dehydration
   c. Cell Shifts: acidemia

Hyperkalemia

1. Are there ECG changes
   a. T Wave peaking
   b. QRS prolongation
2. Recheck the K (is it real?) - it takes a lot longer for a BMP to come back than an ECG
3. Two strategies

There Are ECG Changes			There Aren't ECG Changes		
Stat	IV Calcium	Stabilize Heart			
Temporize	B-agonists Sodium Bicarb Insulin + D50	Reduce Serum K	↓ Total Body K	Kayexalate Furosemide Lots of Volume	↓ K by stool ↓ K by urine ↓K by urine
↓ Total Body K	Kayexalate Furosemide Lots of Volume	↓ K by stool ↓ K by urine ↓K by urine			

Dialysis is always an option. It takes the longest to set up: getting the line, the nephrologist, and the dialysis nurse. Emergently, this is difficult. Start Temporizing and ↓ Total body K measures initially. Don't give lots of volume to someone who doesn't make urine.

134

RENAL NEPHROLOGY KIDNEY

Hypocalcemia

1. Make sure the calcium is actually low
   a. Most exist as albumin bound. The ionized calcium is the calcium that matters, but ionized calcium is an expensive test
   b. For every **1 point of Albumin from 4.0 (normal) add back 0.8 to the reported Calcium**
      i. Total body calcium may be low, but ionized is normal
      ii. If not sure, check an **ionized calcium**
2. Replace Calcium
   a. Give Calcium Gluconate over 1 hour
3. Recognize symptoms
   a. Prolonged QT
   b. Paresthesias, peri-oral tingling, Trousseau sign, Chvostek sign
   c. Hyperventilation induces a temporary and transient hypocalcemic state

Hypercalcemia

1. Spot the symptoms
   a. Kidney Stones
   b. Bones – fractures and bone pain
   c. Groans – abdominal pain, nausea, vomiting, pancreatitis
   d. Psychic Moans – confusion, altered mental status, confusion.
2. Find the cause
   a. All answers (almost) can be answered with **PTH, Phos, Ca, 1,25-Vitamin D**
3. Treat the hypercalcemia
   a. Fluid first. Lots of it. I mean a lot. **NO LASIX**. Give fluid. Lots of it. Have you caught on?
   b. **Calcitonin** (calcium-tone-down) is short lived, but works great for pain
   c. **Alendronate** (bisphosphonates in general) start now, fix them in days
   d. Only give Lasix when they become overloaded. DON'T give diuretics to Hypercalcemic patients. All you'll do is concentrate the serum, making the hypercalcemia worse

Hypophosphate

1. Replete if < 1.0
2. Let them eat if >1.0

Hyperphosphate

1. Renal disease. This is why **phosphate binders** (sevelamer) and **calcimimetics** are added.
2. What you care about is the Ca P product (ca x p). If > 55, you'll have trouble.

CHAPTER 7:   INTERN NOTES

Understanding A Urinalysis

Spec Grav: it's a cheap man's Urine Osms. The higher the spec grav (1.02) the more concentrated the urine. Conversely, the lower the sec grave (1.001) the more dilute.

Protein: if positive, stop doing microalbumin/cr ratios (diabetics) and instead find out how much protein there actually is. Do this with a spot protein to creatinine or 24 hour protein collection (don't do this).

WBC: the more of them there are, the more likely there's an infection.
- 0-5 is normal
- 50-100 is impressive
- > 100 and it's real

Nitrites are made by gram negative rods. They help to suggest infection.

Leukocyte Esterase is made by leukocytes ;). It'll be elevated in an infection.

Squamous Cells: if there are any, ignore the urinalysis and do it again. It means it's contaminated and all you're getting is the stuff from the skin. Clean catch means mid-stream.

Bilirubin: excess bilirubin ends up in the urine.

Urobilinogen: elevation means the biliary duct is **open**.

Glucose: diabetes.

Ketones: DKA, not really good for other kinds. Mild positivity is ignored.

pH: stop looking.

Good sample for UTI

1. Leuk Esterase +
2. Nitrites +
3. WBC > 50
4. Bacteria
5. No Epithelial / Squamous cells

Good sample for DKA

1. Spec Grav 1.020
2. Lots of glucose
3. + Ketones

RENAL NEPHROLOGY KIDNEY

Chronic Kidney Disease

1. Dialysis
   a. Emergent indications (AEIOU)
      i. A: Acidosis
      ii. E: Electrolyte
      iii. I: Ingestion (few things are actually dialyzable)
      iv. O: Overload
      v. U: Uremia
   b. Chronic Indications (GFR Stage)
      i. Stage IV prepare
      ii. Stage V necessary
2. Supporting Urinary Output to Avoid Dialysis
   a. Start with loop diuretic
   b. Add thiazide for synergy
   c. Furosemide + Metolazone is a way to sustain urine output
3. Types of Dialysis
   a. Peritoneal is nightly. It's been gaining favor with nephrologists
   b. Hemo is tiw, requires 4 hours of awake time, and is why there are dialysis centers
4. Inpatient Dialysis Modes
   a. HD: good blood pressure, normal hemodialysis, 3-4 hours
   b. SLED: poor blood pressure, longer to work, 6-12 hours
   c. CVVHD: limited blood pressure, continuous, 24 hours
5. Calcium and Phos
   a. Add Phosphate Binders to keep P low: Sevelamer
   b. Add Calcimimetics to keep PTH low: Cinacalcet
   c. Add Calcium Supplementation to keep PTH low: Calcium Acetate PO
6. HTN
   a. Add ACE or ARB – tolerate 20% rise in Creatinine in 2 weeks
   b. Add CCB
   c. Add Loop diuretics unless they're ESRD (then don't bother)
   d. Add Labetalol
   e. Add Clonidine (the only time you should use clonidine)
   f. Add Minoxidil (you won't add this, Nephrology will)

Kidney Stones

1. Order CT scan without contrast (see stone) or U/S (see hydro)
2. Treat on size, then try to always get a sample of stone

< 5mm	Spontaneous, Fluids, Pain Meds
< 7mm	+ Medical Expulsive Therapy (CCB, alpha-blocker)
< 1.5 cm	Ureteroscopy (distal) Lithotripsy (proximal)
> 1.5 cm	Surgery
Sepsis	Nephrostomy (proximal), Stent (dsital)

NOTES

CHAPTER 7: INTERN NOTES

GI and Liver

Cirrhosis

See common medical conditions

Gi Bleed

1. 2 Large Bore IVs (18 gauge or larger)
2. Type and Cross, Transfuse as needed (H/H serial)
3. Intravenous Fluids (bolus)
4. IV PPI
5. Call GI

See Common medical conditions

Gallbladder

1. Cholelithiasis: colicky abdominal pain with fatty foods. Ultrasound shows gallstones.
2. Cholecystitis: constant pain Ultrasound shows **pericholecystic fluid, gallstones, thickened gallbladder wall**.
   a. Do NOT wait to call surgery → Chole
   b. Abx don't help
3. Choledocolithiasis: Cholecystitis only now with liver enzymes elevated or pancreatitis. Ultrasound shows **dilated ducts**
   a. Do NOT wait to call GI → ERCP
   b. Abx don't help
4. Ascending Cholangitis: Sick as shit choledocolithiasis. Don't waste time with ultrasound - get the ERCP stat
   a. Do NOT wait to call GI → ERCP
   b. Abx <u>do</u> help

Peptic Ulcer Disease

1. Gnawing pain, epigastric, food related (duodenal = after food, gastric = with food)
2. Stop NSAIDs or switch to COX-2, celecoxib
3. H. pylori testing. Treat empirically with triple therapy or quadruple therapy
4. Everyone gets a **PPI**
5. Don't look for Gastrinoma; they're mega rare

138

GI AND LIVER

GERD

1. Retrosternal burning chest pain, worse at night, better with water and antacids
2. "Nocturnal asthma"
3. Empirically treat with PPI, all PPIs are the same (can also use H2 blockers)
4. Scope it if warning symptoms or symptoms persist.
5. Screen once at 5 year, no need to do it again

Ascites

1. Tap it
   a. SAAG $\geq$ 1.1 is good, that's portal hypertension related
   b. SAAG < 1.1 isn't good, that's cancer or TB
   c. >250 polys = SBP --> Ceftriaxone
2. See Common Medical Problems (Cirrhosis)

Ulcerative Colitis

1. Rectal involvement, contiguous lesions, inflammation not outside the colon
   a. Presents as Bloody diarrhea
2. Crypt abscesses and cobblestoning
3. Cancer
   a. First C-scope at 8 years from diagnosis
   b. Annual C-scope there after
   c. Prophylactic Hemicolectomy (also curative of UC)
4. Extraintestinal manifestations
   a. Primary Sclerosing Cholangitis, anterior uveitis, enteropathic arthritis
5. Treatment
   a. 5-ASA compounds (mild)
   b. Steroids (flare)
   c. Colectomy (cure)

Crohn's

1. Intestinal involvement from mouth to anus, skipped lesions
2. Transmural inflammation → fistula formation
3. Treatment
   a. 5-ASA compounds
   b. Infliximab, Rituximab, other biologics
   c. Steroids for flares
   d. Resection not curative

NOTES

CHAPTER 7:   INTERN NOTES

Viral Hepatitis

1. Hep A
   a. Hep A IgM   Active acute infection
   b. Hep A IgG   Vaccine or Immune Exposed
2. Hep B
   a. Hep B s Ag   Active infection
   b. Hep B e Ag   Contagious
   c. Hep B S Ab   Immune; either exposed or vaccinated
   d. Hep B c Ab IGM   Active Infection
   e. Hep B c Ab IGG   Immune; Past exposure only

3. Hep C
   a. Hep C AbChronic Infection

Pancreatitis

1. Make the diagnosis
   a. Lipase elevated = diagnosis
   b. No CT scan at onset (not harmful, just not useful)
2. Treat it
   a. NPO, IV fluids, Pain control (use a PCA pump)
   b. Send labs for Ranson's or Apache II (severity)
   c. Start to feed when the patient is ready
      i. Early refeeding does not help
   d. Do NOT start empiric antibiotics
3. Etiology it = PANCREATITIS, underlined = most common causes

PTH	Rocks (Gallstones)	Infection (mumps)
Alcohol	Estrogen	Triglycerides
Neoplasia	Ace-i	Ischemia (shock)
Calcium	Trauma (ERCP)	Scorpion stings

4. Complications
   a. If the CT scan shows pseudocyst, surgery is > 6 weeks or > 6 cms
   b. If the CT scan shows necrotizing, get a biopsy, treat with Meropenem, necrosectomy weeks later

140

HEME ONC

Heme Onc

Anemia and Transfusions

Transfusion-restrictive strategies generally better.
1. Transfusion Goals
    a. Transfuse to goal of 7.0 in all comers.
    b. Transfuse to goal of 7.0 in variceal hemorrhage, don't go higher
    c. Transfuse to goal of 10 in cardiac patients
    d. Transfuse to achieve asymptomatic condition and to stay ahead of ongoing bleeding (this is a resident level skill)
2. If you're going to transfuse, collect patient's blood first
    a. Microcytic: Ferritin, TIBC, Serum Iron
    b. Macrocytic: B12, Folate, Blood Smear
    c. Normocytic: Reticulocyte count, LDH, Haptoglobin, blood smear

Neutropenic Fever

1. Neutropenia is ANC < 500 (WBC count X % Polys = ANC)
2. Treatment
    a. IV Cefepime
    b. IV Vancomycin if no resolution at day 3
    c. IV Amphotericin if no resolution at day 5
    d. As fever resolves, remove in reverse order, 24 hours at a time
3. Workup
    a. Pan-culture
        i.   CXR
        ii.   UA, Urinalysis
        iii. Blood Cultures
        iv.   C. Diff
    b. Neutropenic Diet, Neutropenic Precautions

NOTES

141

CHAPTER 7:   INTERN NOTES

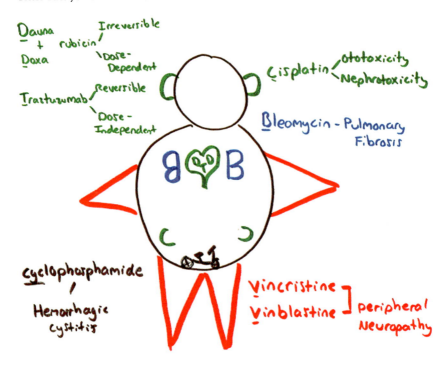

Tumor Lysis Syndrome

Your patient has cancer (cells). You give chemo (cell killer). Cancer cells die. They release uric acid (along with other stuff). That uric acid gets into the kidneys. The kidneys aren't happy and can get seriously injured. The more cells that die (the higher the tumor burden, the higher turnover, and the more susceptible the cancer is) the more likely this is to happen. In particular, look for it with **lymphoma and leukemia**.

1. Prophylaxis:
    a. **Aggressive hydration** (lactated ringers or normal saline). Treat them like rhabdo that hasn't happened yet.
    b. **Allopurinol**
2. Treatment:
    a. Daily creatinine, uric acid
    b. If they start to suffer from Tumor Lysis (even if you did prophylaxis) use **Rasburicase** in addition with large volume resuscitation
    c. If they fluff out because of low urine output and your aggressive hydration, **hemodialysis**.

Heme Onc

Thrombocytopenia

Finding	Dic	TTP
Schistocytes	Yes	Yes
MAHA	Yes	Yes
Low Plts	Yes	Yes
D-Dimer	Elevated	Not Elevated
Fibrinogen	Low	Not low

4Ts For HIT	2	1	0
Timing	5-10 days	After 10	Before 5
Thrombocytopenia	Drop by >50% or Nadir 20	Drop by 30-50% or Nadir 10-20	Drop by <30% or Nadir <10
Thrombosis	New Clot	Progressive Clot	No clot
alTernate	No other cause	Maybe another	Definitely Another

Score	6-8 VERY likely	4-7 MEH likely	0-3 NOT likely
Do...	Treat and get Tests	Get Tests	Do Nothing (for HIT)

Notes

CHAPTER 7: INTERN NOTES

Blood Products

Product	Indications
Blood	Low Hemoglobin, Symptomatic Anemia
Platelets	Thrombocytopenia <20,000 <50,000 and bleeding NOT in TTP / HUS
FFP	Reverse elevated INR
Cryo-precipitate	Decreased Fibrinogen
Massive Transfusion (>3 upRBC in 24 hours)	3 units blood 1 Unit FFP 1 6-pack platelets,monitor ionized Ca
Factors	Multiple factors are in FFP and Cryo. Don't learn them intern year. But white space is provided for you to write it in just in case you encounter a Factor VIII inhibitor patient

Bleeding

1. Causes
   a. Low platelets
   b. Bad platelets
   c. Low factors
   d. Factor inhibitors
2. Workup
   a. CBC (platelets)
   b. PT, PTT, INR with inhibitor study
   c. DON'T order factors (you will on heme, you won't on medicine)
3. Treatment
   a. Low platelets → give platelets (NOT if TTP)
   b. Bad platelets → dialysis (uremia), stop drugs (NSAIDs), ddAVP (vWD)
   c. Low factors → FFP or Factor if known
   d. Inhibitors → Steroids, IVIG, Cyclophosphamide
4. See methods section for more

144

HEME ONC

Transfusion Reactions

1. Transfusion Fever
   a. STOP TRANSFUSION
   b. Give Acetaminophen, Benadryl, but NOT methylprednisolone
   c. Monitor for Hypoxemia, Rash, Airway compromise
   d. If none, may resume the transfusion
2. Anaphylaxis
   a. STOP TRANSFUSION
   b. Send patient's blood and donor blood to lab
   c. Give **Acetaminophen, Benadryl**, and **Methylprednisolone**
   d. Give **epinephrine** if true anaphylaxis (hemodynamic collapse). SubQ first, then as a drip if needed
   e. Intubate if true anaphylaxis (airway collapse). Yes, it's the ABCs and you need to tube early if they're struggling. But, your priority should be on the first 4 unless there's already airway compromise
3. TRALI
   a. STOP TRANSFUSION
   b. Send patient's blood and donor blood to lab
   c. Get a Chest X-ray. You're looking for ARDS
      i. pO2 : FiO2 ratio < 300 (<200 ARDS) → Hypoxemia
      ii. X-ray = fluffy infiltrates
   d. Rule out volume overload (ESRD, CHF) → give Lasix
   e. Give Acetaminophen, Benadryl, Methylprednisolone
   f. Monitor oxygen constantly, intubate early. Sustain with PEEP more than FiO2. CPAP is a great idea if they need more than a venti mask. Don't wait if they're on NRB - impending respiratory failure is around the corner.

NOTES

145

CHAPTER 7:   INTERN NOTES

Sickle Cell Crisis

1. Chronic Pain
   a. This disease hurts. It hurts for the patient's entire life. Your job isn't to "catch" them, "teach them a listen," or "prevent drug abuse." You've never hurt like this patient has and hurt nonstop.
   b. Support them with **as much pain control as they need**. Look at their home regimen to ballpark how much it'll take.
2. Do they have sickle cell disease?
   a. Chronic hemoglobin around 6-8
   b. Chronic reticulocyte count 4-6%
   c. Hgb Electrophoresis to confirm
3. Are they in an acute crisis?
   a. Look at the smear; there should be sickled cells
   b. Look at the Bili; it should be elevated
   c. DON'T look at LDH or Haptoglobin; they're always hemolysing
4. Do they have an emergency?
   a. Priapism
   b. Stroke
   c. Acute Chest
5. Do they have an infection?
   a. Pan culture - CXR, U/A Ux, Blood, and PORTS
   b. Treat if you find something, empiric isn't needed
6. Treat their crisis
   a. **Intravenous fluids**, bolus first and then a rate
   b. **Oxygen** by nasal cannula or as much as they need
   c. Treat infection with antibiotics.
7. Treat their pain
   a. **IV Morphine, Benadryl**, and **Phenergan** does get the patient pretty high (abuse) but it's often what's needed
   b. DON'T withhold pain medications if the patient's awake and in pain
   c. Use a **PCA pump**
      i. Morphine Basal Rate 1mg / hr
      ii. Bolus Rate 1mg / press
      iii. Lockout 15 minutes (4 presses / minute max)
   d. Add IV breakthrough by nursing: **morphine IV** or **dilaudid IV** q4h
   e. Add PO breakthrough by nursing: hydrocodone
   f. Add constipation prophylaxis: Senna 8.6 and Colace 100mg bid

146

HEME ONC

8. Treat their mind

Sometimes patients come in, you find out they're "not in a crisis," and yet here they are. They won't go home. They consume tons of dilaudid and they, "lie about their pain." Very rarely do these people manipulate the system for the sake of manipulation. Take the time to get to know what's happening in their life and WHY they're here. They'll be skeptical of your kindness; they may even think you're trying to catch them in a charade. They'll distrust you. But chip away enough and you'll find the real reason they're in the hospital. If you can help them with their psycho-social stressor, you might just keep them from bouncing back.

NOTES

CHAPTER 7:   INTERN NOTES

Infectious Disease

Urinary Tract Infection

1. Severity
   a. Asymptomatic Bacteriuria → treat only if pregnant
   b. Uncomplicated Cystitis → UTI in a woman without plastic
   c. Complicated Cystitis → UTI in a man, device, or plastic
   d. Pyelonephritis → CVA tenderness, white cell casts
   e. Abscess → CT evidence of abscess formation
2. Treatment
   a. Treat gram negatives
      i.   Ceftriaxone IV or Cipro IV initial therapy.
   b. Obtain culture prior to antibiotics, adjust on sensitivities
   c. Duration is dependent on severity

Uncomplicated	3 days
Complicated	7 days
Pyelo	9 days
Abscess	14 days

3. MKSAP Says
   a. Ambulatory Cystitis → Nitrofurantoin, Bactrim
   b. Ambulatory Pyelo → Cipro
   c. Hospitalized Pyelo → Ceftriaxone

Meningitis

1. LP, CT, Antibiotics
   a. If FAILS positive, give antibiotics, get CT, do puncture
   b. If FAILS negative, get puncture, then antibiotics
2. Empiric antibiotics
   a. Vancomycin IV and Ceftriaxone IV for everyone
   b. Steroids for really sick people
   c. Ampicillin if immunocompromised

Focal Neurologic Deficit
Altered mental status
Immunosuppressed
Lesion over the site of LP
Seizure

148

INFECTIOUS DISEASE

Pneumonia

1. Which is it?
   a. CAP - no exposure to health care
   b. HCAP - exposure to HD, NH, Hospital within 90 days
   c. HAP - pneumonia develops 2 days after admission
   d. VAP - pneumonia develops on a ventilator
2. Make the diagnosis
   a. Fever, Cough, and X-ray findings of consolidation
   b. Sputum cultures rarely help
   c. Blood cultures can be useful
3. Empiric Therapy
   a. Ceftriaxone and Azithromycin for CAP (can do Moxi, but don't)
   b. Vancomycin and Pip.Tazo for everything else
      i. Vanco → Linezolid
      ii. Pip/Tazo → Meropenem

HIV Prophylaxis

CD Count	Bug That Needs Prophylaxis	Prophylaxis Options
CD 4 < 200	PCP	Bactrim Dapsone Atovaquone
CD 4 < 100	Toxo	Bactrim Dapsone Pyrimethamine
CD4 < 50	MAC	Azithromycin weekly

Sulfa allergy = No Bactrim, G6PD deficient = no Dapsone
1. HAART in treatment of HIV (2 + 1)
   a. 2 NRTI + 1 other (determined by genetic studies)
      i. NNRTI
      ii. Protease Inhibitor boosted with Ritonavir
      iii. Integrase Inhibitor
      iv. Entry Inhibitor
      v. Fusion Inhibitor
2. PEP: Post-exposure (rape, condom failure, blood splash, needle stick)
   a. 2+1
3. PrEP: Pre-Exposure Prophylaxis (PrEP)
   a. Truvada = Tenofovir + Emtricitabine (2, not 2 +1)

CHAPTER 7:   INTERN NOTES

Cellulitis

1. Causes
    a.   Staph
    b.   Not Staph
2. Workup
    a.   Rule out dangerous disease with X-ray (Gas Gangrene, Nec Fac, Osteo)
    b.   DON'T MRI every cellulitis
3. Treatment
    a.   Initially IV Vancomycin if in prevalent area
    b.   Transition to oral Bactrim or oral Clinda as cellulitic ring begins to clear
4. Wait... what about clinic
    a.   Try oral2nd generation cephalosporins and assess resolution in a few days.
    b.   If septic, or if treatment failure, admit as above

TB

1. Screening Options
    a.   PPD:
         i.   48-72 hour lag time
         ii.   Do not give if PPD ever positive in life
         iii. Ignore BCG vaccine
    b.   Two tier:
         i.   PPD AGAIN for health care workers
    c.   Interferon Assay, Quantaferon Gold
         i.   One time, One blood test
         ii.   Not available for same day results
    d.   CXR
         i.   If PPD ever positive
         ii.   Annual screen if history of PPD +
    e.   Sputum Samples
         i.   Rule in TB with Sputums q8hx 3
         ii.   Rule out TB with Sputums qAM x 3
2. What if it's not TB?
    a.   MAC is AFB positive, but then cultures weeks later
    b.   Start RIPE, then de-escalate as cultures reveal true organism
3. Treating TB
    a.   Isolate – N95, Droplet precautions
    b.   Use RIPE
    c.   Shorter, Less toxic options becoming available

150

ENDOCRINOLOGY

Endocrinology

Hyperthyroid

1. Presentation = too much "go" signal
   a. Afib / Tachycardia
   b. Diarrhea
   c. Weight Loss
   d. Heat Intolerance
   e. Tremulousness
2. Diagnosis and Causes

All Hyperthyroid will have

↑ T4

↓ TSH

(you won't see secondary hyperthyroidism)

Dz	TSH	T4	RAIU	Thyroglobulin
Graves	↓	↑	Diffuse uptake	↑
Thyroiditis	↓	↑	Cold	↑
Ingestion	↓	↑	Cold	↓
Struma-Ovarii	↓	↑	Cold	↑
Goiter	↓	↑	Nodule	↑

– *Don't take Iodine containing compounds prior to RAIU.*
– *Don't put on PTU or Methimazole prior to RAIU.*
3. Treatment
   a. Beta-blockers for symptom control
   b. If pregnancy not desired = **Radioactive Iodine Ablation**
   c. If pregnancy desired = **PTU** or **Methimazole**
4. Thyroid Storm
   a. Fever, Altered Mental Status, Tachycardia, Shock
   b. Cooling blankets, then Beta-Blockers, PTU / Methimazole, Steroids
   c. Do ablation or surgical resection

Hypothyroid

1. Presentation = too little "go" signal
   a. Bradycardia
   b. Constipation
   c. Weight Gain
   d. Cold Intolerance
2. Diagnosis and Causes
   a. It doesn't matter. If there T4 is low, replace it
   b. T4 ↓, TSH ↑ in most cases (except pituitary deficiency)
3. Treatment
   a. Levothyroxine, test q3 months
   b. If TSH < 10 and no symptoms, don't treat - **subclinical**

Beware "abnormal" thyroid function which is near to baseline in an acutely ill individual. Euthyroid sick syndrome can be sneaky.

151

CHAPTER 7: INTERN NOTES

Cushing's

1. Too much corticosteroids
   a. Diabetes
   b. Hypertension
   c. Dyslipidemia
   d. Obesity (Truncal)
   e. Acne
2. Diagnosis: "Low-Then-high"
   a. Confirm diagnosis with a <u>Low</u>-Dose Dexamethasone suppression test <u>OR</u> 24 hour urinary collection of cortisol
   b. Separate <u>ACTH</u>-dependent from ACTH-independent with an ACTH level
   c. Separate cancer from adrenal function with <u>High</u>-Dose dexamethasone
   d. MRI and Adrenal Vein sampling should also be performed before resection
3. Treatment
   a. Resection

Addison's

1. Too little corticosteroid (death of adrenals or adrenals cannot keep up)
   a. Hypotension
   b. Pressors do not work
   c. Hyperkalemia
2. Diagnosis = Cosyntropin stim test
   a. Baseline cortisol at 8am (must be low to continue)
   b. Cosyntropin 0.25mg at 8am
   c. Cortisol at 830am,900am, 930am
   d. Rise of 20 on the cortisol level indicates SECONDARY adrenal failure

Conn's

1. Too much mineralocorticoid
   a. Hypertension
   b. Hypokalemia
2. Workup
   a. Renin:Aldo ratio (if on Ace or Arb, may have false negative)
   b. Salt load with assessment of aldo
   c. MRI / Adrenal Vein Sampling
3. Treatment
   a. Resection

152

ENDOCRINOLOGY

DKA and HHS (see Common Medical Problems) and HHNK/HHS

DKA is about **D**iabetes (elevated sugar) **K**eto **A**cidosis. HHS doesn't have the K or the A, but it has the D (and the same major problem). The biggest problem is that these patients are dehydrated. Glucose is a potent diuretic. So, unless they have ESRD, DKA or HHS is diagnosed they're **liters behind**.

1. Give Fluids, give a lot of fluids. **Bolus 2-3 Liter of LR, then 200-300cc/hr.** Change to D5½NS when the sugar goes below 250
2. Give Insulin, 10 Units to start, then 0.1 U / kg. Adjust until the rate of glucose decline is about 75/hour
3. Give Potassium,
   a. If K < 3.5 **hold insulin** until you give A LOT of potassium
   b. If K 3.5-5.0, **give potassium and insulin**
   c. If K > 5.0, just watch
4. Follow the K and the Anion Gap (DKA only) with BMP

These are the same diseases except that DKA presents more acutely, less dehydrated, but with more metabolic derangements. HHS presents subacutely taking considerably longer to get dehydrated, but with fewer acid-base problems.

Diabetes Clinic Stuff

1. A1C
   a. > 6.5 % = Diabetes
   b. > 6.0% = preDiabetes
   c. < 6.0% = normal
2. Screening
   a. Retinopathy – retinal screen q1y
   b. Neuropathy – foot exam q1y
   c. Nephropathy – urinalysis q1y
3. Treatment
   a. Orals first – Metformin, Glipizide, … other expensive stuff you shouldn't use
   b. Insulins after 2 orals fail
      i. Start Basal, titrate fasting sugar
      ii. Add Bolus, prandial
      iii. Goal is qAc and qHs

CHAPTER 7:   INTERN NOTES

Rheumatology

Serology

Serology	Disease	Serology	Disease
ANA	Gateway lab	Ro	Sjogren's
RF	Gateway Lab	La	Sjogren's
dsDNA	r/i Lupus	Scl-70	Scleroderma
Smith	r/i Lupus	Centromere	CREST
Histone	r/i Drug Induced Lupus	ANCA	Wegener's

Arthrocentesis

	Osteoarthritis	Inflammatory	Septic
Wbc	<5,000	5,000-50,000	>50,000
Fluid	Serous (See through)	Cloudy	White, Turbid
Stain	Nothing	Crystals	Organisms

Lupus

MDSOAP BRAIN

Malar Rash	**B**lood
Discoid Rash	**R**enal
	ANA
Serositis	**I**mmunologic
Oral Ulcers	**N**eurologic
Arthritis	
Photosensitivity	

Lupus Joints: Hydroxychloroquine > Methotrexate
Lupus Flare: IV Methylprednisolone → Oral prednisone
Nephritis: Cyclophosphamide

Infection vs Flare

	Infection	Flare
Complement	C3/4 Normal	Reduced C3/4
dsDNA	Normal	Elevated
Leukocytosis	Elevated	Normal

154

RHEUMATOLOGY

Rheumatoid Arthritis

Nobody Should Have RA Symptoms 3 times (X)
N odules
S ymmetric
H ands - MCP/PIP
R F or CCP
S tiffness (>1 hour)
3 joints or more involved
X -ray findings (erosions)

Chronic Disease: Methotrexate > Hydroxychloroquine
Escalate Therapy: Biologic + Methotrexate
Pain control: NSAIDs -- never as monotherapy

Seronegatives (Pair)

Psoriasis - rash and arthritis (arthritis may precede rash)
Ank Spond - low back pain
IBD-related (enteropathic) - UC/Crohn's and arthritis
Reactive - arthritis and STDs (Reiter)

Scleroderma And Crest

Calcinosis	CREST
Reynaud's	Kidneys
Esophageal Dysmotility (GERD)	Lungs
Sclerodactyly	Hear
Telangiectasias	

NO pulmonary disease but	YES pulmonary disease and
YES pulmonary hypertension	YES pulmonary hypertension
Centromeres	Topoisomerase / scl-70

NOTES

CHAPTER 7:   INTERN NOTES

Gout And Pseudogout

1. Diagnosis
   a. Gout need shaped negative birefringent
   b. Pseudogout rhomboid shaped positively birefringent
2. Treatment, Flare
   a. Colchicine if unable to give NSAIDs (renal disease)
   b. Steroids if they don't work / can't give
3. Treatment, Chronic (if more than 1 attack / 6 month, goal Uric Acid < 7.0)
   a. Allopurinol
      i. Don't start during flare
      ii. May precipitate flare
      iii. Continue through flare, use NSAID / Colchicine / Steroids as above
   b. Stop Thiazides
   c. Stop Red Wine
   d. Stop Red Meat
   e. Stop Known Precipitants (Crawfish)

Hardly anyone responds to probenecid – don't use it

NEURO

Neuro

Stroke

See common medical problems

Seizure

1. Is it status epilepticus?
   a. **Ongoing seizures or no return to baseline for 20 minutes**
      i. Give Ativan, Ativan, Ativan, and Ativan
      ii. Fosphenytoin load
      iii. Midazolam and Propofol (intubate here)
      iv. Phenobarbital
2. Why are they seizing?
   a. VITAMINS

Vascular	**M**etabolic
Infection	**I**ngestion / Withdrawal
Trauma	**N**eoplasm
Autoimmune	**S**omething else (medication noncompliance)

3. Treat their seizure
   a. **Increase** the dose or add an agent
      i. **Keppra**
      ii. Phenytoin
      iii. Valproate

Weakness

See Methods
Characterize the location of the weakness and the likely area affected.

Headache

See Methods
Don't scan everyone. CT for secondary causes of headache. Symptomatic treatment of primary headache.

Back Pain

See Methods
Image very few patients. Image people who have focal neurologic deficits or in which cord compression syndrome is suspected. Secondary causes of back pain need imaging and intervention. Most causes of back pain need Flexeril.

NOTES

157

ICU

Ahhhhhh!

Teh Unitz!!

I am so scurred!

Chill.

The unit is easier than you think.

Let's give you the tools to dominate here.

FIRST RULE:

Do no harm.

CHAPTER 8: ICU

Sick, Not Sick, On the Fence

<u>The most important skill an PGY-1 learns is to identify sick vs not sick.</u>

The goal of this lesson is to enable you to determine just how sick someone is **without** even considering the patient's story, labs, diagnosis, etc. This assessment should be able to be done by **looking at the numbers alone**. With experience, you'll start to feel how sick someone is when you walk into the room. That initial impression will start to make sense. To help get you there, start with a **concrete** method for approaching vital signs. This will also allow you to reflect on the impression you have - do the numbers line up with what you're feeling?

As you **start PGY-1**, you want your spectrum to look like this:

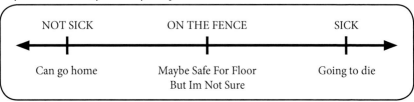

As you **finish PGY-1**, you want your spectrum to look like this:

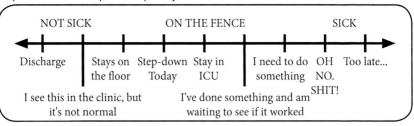

As you **finish PGY-3**, you want your spectrum to look like this:

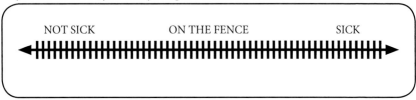

You may already be able to do this a little. Let's see:

HR 65   Ok   HR 180   WHAT!? 180!? IS THAT POSSIBLE
HR 102 Well that's not normal   HR 220   <deer in headlights>
HR 135 Whoa, cool - 135

160

SICK, NOT SICK, ON THE FENCE

This is what you should do with every patient every time.

Look at the numbers: the **cardiovascular system** (heart rate and blood pressure), the **respiratory system** (oxygenation, pulse Ox; ventilation, respiratory rate) and the **nervous system** (level of consciousness).

You should make an assessment on the **number alone**. Just look at the monitor and evaluate. DON'T take into consideration the patient's condition, diagnosis, or history. Just focus on the numbers.

Then, you should **contextualize the number** by looking at the **medication tower** or the **ventilator**. Again, no history, diagnosis, or story - just the numbers and the medications being used to support them.

This skill is particularly useful in **daily ICU assessments** and the **day of admission** when you see the person for the first time in the ED. It's something the ED does really well. You need to learn to do it better so you can be the one to make the right disposition decision.

1. Cardiovascular System
    a. Heart Rate
        Look at the **heart** rate. Sick, not sick, on the fence.
        Look at the **medication tower**. Are there meds that change the degree of illness?
    b. Blood Pressure
        Look at the **blood pressure** (the MAP). Sick, not sick, on the fence.
        Look at **the medication tower.** Are there meds that change the degree of illness?
2. Pulmonary system
    a. Oxygenation
        Look at the **pulse ox**. Sick, not sick on the fence.
        Look at the **ventilator**. How much oxygen / PEEP do they require to get there?
    b. Ventilation
        Look at the **respiratory rate**. Sick, not sick, on the fence.
        Look at the **ventilator**. What is the peak pressure, tidal volumes?
3. Nervous System
    a. AMS
        Are they **altered, lethargic**, or **combative**?
        Look at the **medication tower**. Are there meds that change the degree of illness?

By the way: YOU decide, in your soul and inside yourself, what "sick" means. There are some things most people agree on, but YOU make that call. There isn't a magic cut-off for any value.

161

CHAPTER 8: ICU

Who Goes to the Unit?

For some people it's OBVIOUS they need the unit. There's the guy who is frankly hypotensive already on pressors or the guy who already on the ventilator. That's not the point. That's obvious even to a medical student. You want to get a gestalt for who is and isn't sick. BUT, if something concrete can be used to start that process, ie some objective data, wouldn't that be cool?

Pulmonary Embolism

Diagnosis	Symptoms	Heart Strain	Vitals	Location
Asymptomatic PE	No	No	Floor	Home
Symptomatic PE	Yes	No	Floor	Floor
Submassive PE	Yes	Yes	Unit	Unit
Massive PE	Yes	Yes	Unit	**Unit**

GI Bleed:
Who: Orthostatics
Why: Fluids, Blood, Nursing

Sepsis/Septic Shock

Stroke:
tPA → Unit
worsening stroke → Unit
Hemorrhagic → Unit
Needs q1h neurocheck

Diagnosis	How to make the call	Location
Sepsis	2/4 SIRS criteria + a source	Home
Severe Sepsis	Hypotension responsive to fluid lactated clears. ~2Liters	Floor
Septic Shock	Hypotension Unresponsive to fluid. Lactate fails to clear. Pressors	Unit
Multiorgan Failure	All organs in dysfunction. This person is probably going to die.	Unit

COPD / Asthma:
Rising CO2
Decreasing breath sounds
Inadequate response of
FEV1

DKA:
If there's D K and A go to the unit. Some can be handled on the floor. Why bother?

Hepatic Encephalopathy

Stage	Sxs	Asterixis	Dispo
I	Mild cognitive impairment, memory	No	Floor
II	Altered, but still saying real words	Yes	Floor
III	Incomprehensible Sounds, Moaning	Yes	Unit
IV	Coma	No (can't)	Unit

162

ARDS - Lung Protective Strategy

Ventilation

The normal lung has equal distribution of pressure throughout it. This is because there's **homogeneity**. When there's ARDS, the lung goes towards **heterogeneity**. Whichever part of the lung is dependent becomes **concrete**, which harms the lung's ability to ventilate. So, when a lot of pressure is pushed into the lung, only the normal lung gets ventilated; the ARDS lung doesn't. SOOOOO, ALL the pressure goes towards the good lung, causing it to get stretched. That means **more inflammation and worse ARDS**. Push too hard and you get a pneumothorax. Keeping pressures low (see Oxygen delivery) requires **low Tidal Volumes**.

Oxygenation

Part of the problem with ARDS is an abundance of fluid. The capillaries get leaky, so the fluid not only creates a **diffusion barrier** (limits oxygen diffusion), but more importantly, it collapses alveoli and prevents them from opening back up. This is called **de-recruitment**. In ARDS, the lung can't really be **de-recruited** until the ARDS is gone.

Thus, the goal's to **prevent de-recruitment**. Do so by maintaining **high PEEP**.

This does two things. It prevents de-recruitment (which is huge), but it also increases oxygen delivery to the blood.

Avoid high FiO2 if possible, because long term oxygen delivery leads to worsening pulmonary fibrosis.

What I want you to take away from this is: **use PEEP, not FiO2. Use RR, not Tv.**

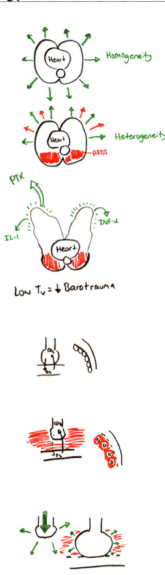

CHAPTER 8:   ICU

Ventilator Strategy

Initial Settings VC	
RR	15
Tv	500
PEEP	5
FiO2	100%

Oxygen Delivery

See the spectrum of oxygen delivery modes. The lowest is room air. Each oxygen delivery method requires more liters per minute to work. But they also provide more FiO2 per liter per minute. **Nasal cannula** works on 1-6 LPM; it adds about 2% FiO2 per LPM. **Non-rebreathers** (NRB) provide (theoretically) 100% FiO2, but, because there's no seal, only reach about 80%.

When in a pinch, just start at a non-rebreather, then de-escalate downwards if they maintain their sat at 100%. If necessary, escalate to more invasive modes oxygenation goals.

ICU level modes happen once there's a need for more oxygen than that delivered by NRB. It begins with **noninvasive positive pressure ventilation**, which comes in the form of CPAP, High Flow Nasal Cannula (theoretically equal to CPAP), and BiPAP.
The most advanced, invasive, and best oxygen delivery mode available is the **endotracheal tube**.

Monitoring Gases

There are two gases you care about. **Oxygen** represents **oxygenation** (duh). **Carbon Dioxide** represents **ventilation**.

Oxygen can be measured with either the **pulse oximeter** or the **arterial blood gas**. If there's a good wave form you DON'T need to get an ABG. If you're getting an ABG for oxygen, think about doing something else.

Carbon dioxide is measured only by **arterial blood gas**. If tracking CO2, an ABG is NEEDED to do it.

Adjusting Gases

Oxygen can be **increased** by **upping** either the **PEEP** or the **FiO2**.

Carbon dioxide can be **decreased** by **increasing** either **respiratory rate, tidal volume**, or **PsOP** (bipap). PsOP on bipap is known as "iPap, or inspiratory pressure".

164

Ventilator Strategy

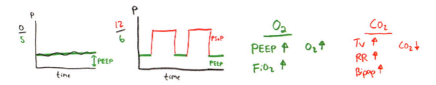

NIPPV Modes

CPAP is all about **PEEP**. It's reported as 0/X, where X is a number. When you say "CPAP 5" you mean "PEEP 5." PEEP is **positive end expiratory pressure** and helps retain recruitment of alveoli. That's good for oxygen delivery. The FiO2 can also be set in addition to PEEP.

BiPAP has PEEP built in; it's still the bottom number. But BiPAP does something pretty cool. It also gives an inspiratory pressure, which I refer to as the Pressure Support over Peep (PSoP). There's always a little PEEP, but then with each breath more pressure is added on inspiration, then cut off on exhalation. The machine works with the patient. To use BiPap the patient needs to be **alert, not vomiting**, and **working with the machine**. It's reported as Y/X, such as, "BiPap, 12 / 6." That means there's always a PEEP of 6, but with each inhalation, give a little extra puff to bring them to 12. This is good for **ventilation**.

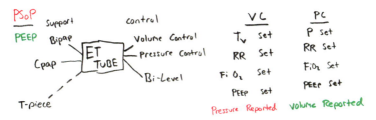

ET Tubes

This is its own section. **Support modes** are just like NIPPV: they don't have a set respiratory rate and the machine waits for the patient to breathe to activate. In support modes, PEEP of 5 "is the resistance of the machine" and approximates room air. The **spontaneous breathing trial** is 0/5, meaning "CPAP at peep of 5." Do an SBT every day (at least once).

Control modes take over for the patient, that is, the machine breathes for them. You set the rate, the PEEP, the FiO2, and other thing that's mode dependent. In **volume control mode**, set the tidal volume. The machine gives it and **tells the pressure** it took to give that volume. Conversely, in pressure control mode set the pressure. The machine gives it and **tells the volume** you were able to get. I like volume control modes because I know how to adjust the machine to reduce the pressure (Tv down, respiratory rate up - see ARDS and lung protective strategies).

| Goal: Ppeak < 30 | SpO2 95-98% | pCO2 < 40 | PEEP and FiO2 as low as possible |

CHAPTER 8: ICU

Common Medications in the ICU: Sedation and Paralysis

Sedation

Infusions	
Propofol (Diprivan)	Rapid on and rapid off **Drops Blood Pressure**, drops respiratory rate Can cause Propofol infusion syndrome if used for long term
Dexmedetomidine (Precedex)	Propofol alternative **No change in blood pressure**, no change in respiratory rate Can be used for alcohol withdrawal
Fentanyl	**Pain control** Does nothing to Blood Pressure 1st line agent for ventilated patients
Pushes	
Lorazepam	Because you want them to be quiet Alcohol withdrawal
Midazolam	Status Epilepticus. Don't use this otherwise
Etomidate	Used in RSI with rocuronium vs vecuronium. Don't use this otherwise

DON'T USE ATIVAN AS A DRIP. YOU'LL STACK THE DOSE AND THEY WON'T WAKE UP. Use q2 or q4h scheduled pushes, but NOT a drip.

Paralysis

Pushes (Rapid Sequence Paralytics)	
Succinylcholine	Depolarizing agent (**Check the K, don't give if K is elevated**) 1mg/kg given with Etomidate 3mg/kg for RSI
Rocuronium	Nondepolarizing agent (**Use when you can't use Succs**) 1mg/kg given with Etomidate 3mg/kg for RSI

Infusions (Paralytics Used In Ards)	
Cisatracurium	When they're so sick that they need to be paralyzed on the ventilator (their ARDS is so bad). They probably have organ dysfunction, so use this
Vecuronium	Don't use this

166

Common Medications in the ICU: Sedation and Paralysis

RSI	Intubated Patients	ARDS + ↑ PPeak	Status Epilepticus
Etomidate 3mg/kg	Fentanyl	Cisatracurium	Midazolam
And	And	(aka paralyze)	And propofol
Succs 1mg/kg (K ok)	Propofol (BP ok)		
Or	Or		
Roc 1mg/kg (K high)	Precedex (BP not ok)		

Picking which sedation to use isn't hard. Often, when someone is intubated you'll be dealing with more than just their airway. That is, if there's simultaneous circulatory compromise, there must be a tenuous balance between getting their pressure up and improving their breathing.

We use sedation **while intubated** to make it more comfortable for the patient (fentanyl because the tube hurts) and to help them not fight the tube. **Always do this**, unless the patient happens to be trached and ventilated.

We use paralysis **while intubated** to reduce airway pressures. The only time this happens is in ARDS. IE the FiO2 and PEEP have both been maxed out, yet their Ppeaks are still in the 40s with plateau pressure still in the high 30s. Paralysis is given just before you start prone positioning. This will **rarely happen** and you'll likely **never do it on your own**.

Every shift the nurses will **turn off sedation** and attempt a **spontaneous breathing trial**. Make sure this is ordered for at least daily, if not every shift. The sedation comes off to see how they do on the ventilator and how they do without sedation. Having no sedation is cruel and unusual, but a calm person who doesn't move off sedation is probably dead, while someone staring at you pointing at the tube with the gesture of "get this out of my throat" is probably doing well. Please try to be **at the bedside** when they do the awakening trial, if possible.

CHAPTER 8: ICU

In the ICU: Approach to Shock

Shock is about poor tissue perfusion. What you will refer to, in about 99.99% of cases, is **low blood pressure**. But I want you to change your lingo. You're in the Unit, and so the vocabulary should adjust accordingly.

The **only thing that matters for perfusion is the MAP**

Don't say blood pressure. Don't say "Some Number Over Some Number." In the unit, the words "systolic" and "diastolic" shall not be uttered. Say "the map is…"

So, when encountering someone with a **decreased mean arterial pressure (MAP)**

DRAW THIS OUT. EVERY. TIME.

Don't skip. Consider all components, working your way around the equation.

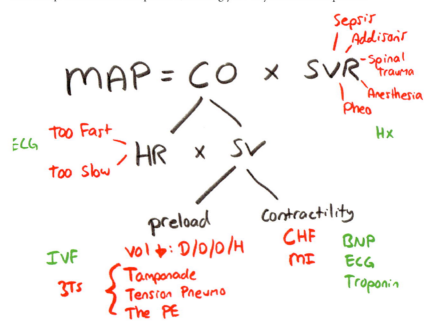

IN THE ICU: APPROACH TO SHOCK

1. **Heart Rate**: it's either too slow or too fast. You must first ensure that is not compensatory by getting an **ECG**. If it's **sinus tach** you haven't found the culprit; the search continues for the physiologic stressor. Otherwise, because they're in shock, **Pace slow rhythms, shock fast ones**.
2. Preload: preload comes in two forms.
    a. The first is volume depletion as occurs in the "4Ds" **Diarrhea, Dehydration, Diuresis**, and **Hemorrhage** (ok, the last one isn't a D). This will respond with volume expansion.
    b. The second is **obstruction** which means the **Tension Pneumo, Tamponade**, and **The PE** (to make the Three Ts work). These will initially respond to fluids but some other intervention is ultimately required.
3. **Contractility**
    a. **CHF** or **MI**. Use the **BNP** and the **Bedside Sonogram** to assess ejection fraction. Support with inotropes and revascularize if that's the issue
4. **SVR**
    a. The list is long, with interventions dependent on the underlying cause. Look for **sepsis, anaphylaxis, Addison's disease, spinal trauma, epidural anesthesia**, and for some reason, pheochromocytoma (this happened once, so I now include it). Ultimately, the goal will be to replace the systemic vascular resistance with a vaso-constrictive medication, but which one you pick is dependent on the underlying diagnosis.

Cardiac output versus Systemic Vascular resistance

The **Blood Pressure (MAP)** is supported by both **cardiac output** and by **systemic vascular resistance**. If one goes down, the other will go up. Since cardiac output is comprised of Heart Rate, Preload, and Contractility, if one goes down the others will also increase.

That means the first thing to do is determine if the shock in front of you is a problem with **SVR** or **CO**. I want you to see **SVR** as diastolic tone and **CO** as systolic whomp. Ok, so if the CO goes down there'll be little systemic whomp. But SVR will increase in order to keep the MAP up. Diastolic tone also goes up. That'll result in less perfusion to the distal extremities (**cold wrists and ankles** - don't use hands or feet as those autoregulate differently). Also, since we've lost systolic whomp the **pulse pressure narrows**.

Conversely, if the SVR goes down there'll be a loss of diastolic tone. The peripheral vasculature opens up and blood flows. This means there will be **warm wrists and ankles** despite low blood pressure. The systolic whomp is still intact (systolic stays high) while the diastolic tones falls, leading to a **widened pulse pressure**.

Of course, the history and leading diagnosis are best in determining what's wrong, but as a starting point, figure out if it is CO or SVR.

CHAPTER 8:   ICU

Obvious and Hidden Shock

	Heart Rate	Blood Pressure	Shock Index	
Shock Index	86	112/86	0.76	No problem
	130	110/62	1.18	Uh oh
Occult Shock	Clinic 4 months ago	Clinic 4 weeks ago	Now in ED	
	160/110 4 meds	158/96 4 meds	120/80 no meds	
Frank Shock	Map < 65			

But how can you tell if there's shock at all? When the MAP is less than 65 there's **frank shock**. Most people get that pretty easy. The blood pressure is low. Done. But there are types of shock that are commonly missed.

A shock index is when the **heart rate is greater than the systolic blood pressure**. It's associated with an elevated lactate, which in turn is indicative of a worse mortality. This has to be taken into context, of course. The maximum heart rate is 220-age. A young woman in her 20s with pyelonephritis and no history of hypertension may be in the 130s heart rate, have a blood pressure of 96/46 (her normal), and be totally fine. Meanwhile, the 70 year old on anti-hypertensives in the same situation is in trouble. Much like the SIRS criteria, the idea is that a shock index doesn't guarantee sick, but if identified there should be extra thought put into the patient.

Occult Shock occurs when the MAP is greater than 65 but there's still poor tissue perfusion. This happens in patients who have chronically elevated MAPs. They're "used to" living at 180/100, and so 120/60 is actually low for them.

Lactic acidosis. An elevated lactate means **poor tissue perfusion**. It DOESN'T mean sepsis or shock, only that tissue is dying. An elevated lactate should immediately bump someone up to higher acuity. A failure of the lactic acid to clear with intervention gets that person an admission to the unit.

170

In the ICU: Pressors

Choosing pressors isn't too hard. It becomes so when you try to remember all the dosages (how many mcg/kg/ min) and how many "+" signs are in each receptor type. Instead, sit back, make a diagnosis, then choose the pressor to go with the diagnosis. This will take courage, since you'll know what's going to happen (or what you want to happen) and the nurses are going to have only their own personal experience. You'll often have to insist on which pressor you pick. But, as long as you know WHY you're picking it, you must be steadfast in your decision.

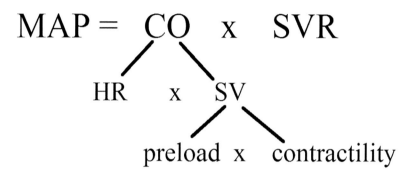

Vasoconstrictors	Inoconstrictors	Inodilators	Vasodilators
Vasopressin	Levophed (Norepi)	Dobutamine	Cardene
Epinephrine	Dopamine	Milrinone	Nitric Oxide
Phenylephrine			Esmolol
SVR shock	Septic Shock	CHF	HTN emergency

Indication to Pressor

Septic Shock	Cardiogenic Shock	Anesthesia, Spinal	Anaphylaxis
1. Levo or Dopa	Dobutamine	Phenylephrine	Epinephrine
2. Vasopressin	+/- Dopa		
3. STEROIDS		GI Bleed	PE
4. Epinephrine	Milrinone	BLOOD	tPA
Pick up the phone	+/- Levo	FLUIDS	

Arrhythmia? ELECTRICITY

CHAPTER 8: ICU

In the ICU: Septic Shock

Fluid

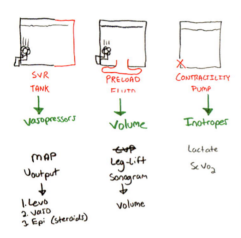

When sepsis is diagnosed the patient is volume down. But when it comes to how much fluid to give, the jury's still out. The most progressive you can be is to **restrict volume** (2-3 liters) and use **lactated ringers**. If the MAP isn't at goal after 3 liters, just start pressors.

Volume restriction will reduce the risk of ARDS. If they're dumped with fluid, their capillaries open up - all that fluid you just gave ends up in their lungs. That's not good; it worsens ARDS and has poor outcomes. Stop dumping 6-7 liters into someone with sepsis.

Lactated ringers is preferred over Normal Saline because it produces no acidosis. It's also pH neutral so it won't worsen an underlying acidosis, which is already bad. Since you won't be giving a large volume resuscitation anymore, it really doesn't matter, but also please stop giving saline and start giving ringers to just about everyone.

Assessing adequate volume resuscitation is really freaking hard. First, you have to ensure you've resuscitated and daily requirements are continued to be provided. Get the number close. Luckily, there are a few tools to help in deciding whether additional boluses will be useful:

1. **CVP:** Useless. It requires zero skill to use, but also doesn't yield anything you don't already know. This has been repeatedly shown to be bogus. Don't use CVPs.
2. **Bedside Echo:** Requires some skill here. What to look for is the IVC located at the level of the liver. If it collapses with each heartbeat the person is volume down; they need fluid.
3. **Leg Lift – Art Line:** An arterial line is needed for this. With your partner, perform a leg lift (you literally just lift the legs), which effectively delivers a fluid bolus from stagnant fluid in the veins of the legs. If the blood pressure increases (MAP ~10 ↑) they need fluid.

Fluid assessment is a multiple-time-per-day kind of thing. The goal is to sustain preload while not overloading the pulmonary system.

IN THE ICU: SEPTIC SHOCK

Pressors

Dopamine = Levophed, so if the ED starts Dopamine there's no need to change it. But there's a very specific and tested order in which you add pressors.

Levophed, then **Vasopressin**, then **Steroids** (adrenal insufficiency), then **epinephrine**. In all honesty, if you have to start epinephrine the next move is likely **picking up the phone** to call the family about discontinuation.

DON'T GIVE BICARB. It's the marker of death. Have the courage to let a dying patient die, the strength to help a grieving family grieve.

Intubation

The diaphragm can consume up to 20% of the cardiac output. Because SVR is compromised, the delivery of oxygen to the distal tissues is compromised. That elevated lactate means tissue is dying. If you instead **paralyze and sedate** the patient, the ventilator does the work the diaphragm was doing. Boom, free oxygen delivery that would have gone to the diaphragm now goes everywhere else.

If starting a pressor for septic shock, give some serious thought as to why you SHOULDN'T intubate that patient. In the absence of overwhelming reasons against **intubation you should reflex to intubating all septic shock patients**.

Other stuff with less evidence (aka things aren't going well so let's try something)

Blood

Probably not ever indicated in a sepsis unless there's also hemorrhage or DIC. BUT, theoretically, if there's a **persistently elevated lactate** AND **Low ScVO2** AND Anemia then maybe, MAYBE the patient could benefit from blood. There's definitely no need for albumin or plasma.

Inotropes

Usually the cardiac system picks up speed when SVR is compromised. Contractility and heart rate go up in response to a decreased SVR. BUT, just like blood, if there's a **persistently elevated lactate** AND **Low ScVO2** AND **Depressed Cardiac Function**, then maybe, MAYBE the patient could benefit from inotropes (though usually it just causes tachyarrhythmias).

CHAPTER 8: ICU

In the ICU: Running a Code

Running a code is more about **herding cats** than it is medicine. Here, your goal as the doctor is to act as **team leader**. Act and speak with confidence. Assign roles. Control the team or they'll control you.

Walk into the room and say out loud, *"who is in charge of this code?"* Then stare at the person you think is in charge. If no one responds, **take command**. "Dustyn for the code, Dr. Williams for the chart." If someone responds, ask them **if they need help**. Then either take over or step back and get out of their way. "Dr. Lee has control of the code."

Assign roles to everyone in the code. "I know you know how to run a code. Let me give you a role so you know what to do in THIS code."

Speak out loud and **plan the next 6 minutes**. People will be impressed. That gives them confidence in you. They'll listen to you. Loud, chaotic codes are your fault - not the nurses.

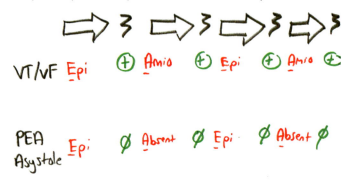

The code:

A code is built upon **2 minute blocks of CPR**. Whether that's five cycles of 30 compressions to 2 ventilations or just 2 minutes of continuous compressions, all codes are blocked in 2 minute intervals.

Each 2 minute block = **1 medication, 1 pulse check, 1 rhythm check**, and **1 shock if indicated**.
There are two types of rhythms, and so two types of codes:

1. Vtach / Vifb: use **epi** alternating with **amio** and you **can shock**
2. PEA / Asystole: use **epi** alternating with **nothing** and you **can't shock**

That's it. Go for **12 minutes**. Then **ask everyone** if they want to continue or have any ideas. Unless you know they're acidotic or have hyperkalemia, **DON'T GIVE BICARB**.
Compressions are more important than lines, intubations, and medications

In the ICU: Running a Rapid

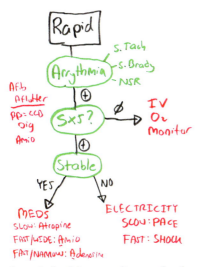

When the patient **has a pulse** things are a lot harder; it's far less algorithmic. Regardless of the complaint or the reason you were called, an approach to that problem is needed (see methods section). For this discussion, we're assuming there's a **cardiac rapid response**. In any rapid you have to act. But also be ok with thinking, with silence, and with asking for more information.

Begin by assessing **how sick they are**. If more resources are needed, a line has to be put in, or you have to intubate, do it. If the patient needs to be moved to the unit, ensure they're stable enough to do so. You have 5-7 people in a rapid in the room, 2 people in the elevator.

Step 1: Is this a cardiac arrhythmia problem? For the sake of this discussion the answer is yes. Sinus Tach, **Sinus Brady and Normal Sinus Rhythm AREN'T ARRYTHMIAS.**

Step 2: Are there symptoms? If no symptoms, **start an IV** (in case you have to intervene), give them **Oxygen** (doesn't hurt acutely), and put them on tele, a **heart monitor**.

Step 3: Are they stable? No. **Stability** is defined by your comfort level. Some will consider anything not-dead (a code) to be stable. That isn't wrong. As you start, see the AHA definition of **MAP < 90**, or **AMS /CP / SOB** associated with onset of arrhythmia as unstable. From there, your comfort zone will subsequently grow.

In an unstable patient, there's no time to play. You must intervene RIGHT NOW or they'll die. That means **electricity**.
    a. **Unstable + Fast = Shock**
    b. **Unstable + Slow = Pace**

Step 3: Are they stable? Yes. Now there's time to stay and play. To get the IV access. To wait for meds from pharmacy. Something needs to be done but there are minutes of freedom.
    a. Stable + Slow = Atropine, prepare to pace
    b. Stable + Fast + Wide = Amiodarone
    c. Stable + Fast + Narrow = Adenosine
    d. Stable + Fast + Afib/Flutter = CCB or BB. Adenosine will not hurt (it won't help either)

Personal Notes

Personal Notes

Personal Notes